Nurses, Computers and Information Technology

Nurses, Computers and Information Technology

Paula M. Procter

PMP Communications, Sheffield, UK

CHAPMAN & HALL

London · Glasgow · New York · Tokyo · Melbourne · Madras

Published by Chapman & Hall, 2–6 Boundary Row, London SE1 8HN

Chapman & Hall, 2–6 Boundary Row, London SE1 8HN, UK

Blackie Academic & Professional, Wester Cleddens Road, Bishopbriggs, Glasgow G64 2NZ, UK

Chapman & Hall, 29 West 35th Street, New York, NY10001, USA

Chapman & Hall Japan, Thomson Publishing Japan, Hirakawacho Nemoto Building, 6F, 1–7–11 Hirakawa-cho, Chiyoda-ku, Tokyo 102, Japan

Chapman & Hall Australia, Thomas Nelson Australia, 102 Dodds Street, South Melbourne, Victoria 3205, Australia

Chapman & Hall India, R. Seshadri, 32 Second Main Road, CIT East, Madras 600 035, India

Distributed in the USA and Canada by Singular Publishing Group Inc., 4284 41st Street, San Diego, California 92105

First edition 1992

© 1992 Chapman & Hall

Phototypeset in 10/12pt Palatino by Intype, London
Printed in Great Britain by St Edmundsbury Press,
Bury St Edmunds, Suffolk

ISBN 0 412 33450 X   1 56593 019 3 (USA)

A catalogue record for this book is available from the British Library

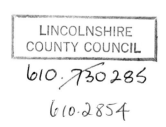

Contents

Acknowledgements

It is always difficult to acknowledge all those who have been instrumental in one's professional development. There are some who stand out and others who appear upon immediate reflection to have had less significant influence, yet their support, knowledge and encouragement have been vital to that development.

I thank my father for accepting that even as a child I investigated how mechanical objects worked, thus forming the cornerstone to my later interest in technology, and also for his support and guidance throughout the production of the text for this book.

From a nursing perspective, I would like to thank Jean Jarvis for encouraging my first steps into the world of nurses, computers and information technology, and for her continued support as my career developed. My thanks also go to Barbara Rivett, through whose guidance my eyes were opened to the implications of technology upon nursing; to David Jones, who saw the potential for national educational development of computers and information technology and allowed me to supervise such a development; and to the ENB CAL Project team, Sandy Massie, Margaret Jupe, Phillip Russell-Lacy, Pam Brand, Paul Turner, Catherine Waller, Stella Shailer and Mike James, and Helen Betts as an associate team member, for their enthusiasm, dedication and support during the project. All those I have met during my travels who challenged, questioned, agreed and disagreed during discussions both long and short, I thank you for your scepticism which helped me to rationalize directions taken, and for your motivation, which spurred my professional development and indeed the writing of this book.

Preface

Another book about computers; well yes, but with no apology for its production. This book is for those with a lot of nursing knowledge and little or no computer knowledge. Indeed, it is suitable for anyone in the nursing, midwifery or health visiting arena, for it takes its base from what is known to all.

What is known is our role in our chosen health care profession. What is unknown and requires development is the potential for each of us to think constructively about the role a computer could play in our working environment, be that education or clinical practice.

This is not a technical book. My intention is to give sufficient information to readers to motivate them to have a go at using a computer. If you fall into the category of an interested person not quite knowing where to start, then this could be the book for you!

I have developed greater knowledge with certain computers than others but, to enhance this publication, I have used a variety of computer types, programs and applications, so that very few stones have been left unturned; indeed only small pebbles are left. Once you have browsed, or even worked through the book, it could be expected that you would have enough knowledge to move on to one of the more sophisticated texts on the market and be in a position to understand the potential power of computers and information technology for nursing.

Chapter One

Why nurses should concern themselves with computers

Health care has always been a part of general society which has moved, over the generations, through many different developmental stages to attain the post-industrial arena of today. As each of us relates only to one generation within the movement it is sometimes difficult to comprehend the changes taking place and the speed of such changes.

Present-day society is moving faster technologically than any previous age. Many argue that the technological revolution has accelerated beyond man's wildest dreams. We must now begin the process of education for technology in order that we may understand our potential capabilities in readiness for the next move forward.

It is the aim of this book to assist in that educational process; the main area of the book's concern is that of assisting in building the required general understanding of computer and information technology within the nursing* framework.

WHY USE COMPUTERS?

The first question to be asked is why nurses should concern themselves with computers, for if nurses do not need to know about computers and information technology then it is not necessary to go beyond this line. However, it is possible that the question merits further analysis, especially in the changing nature of nursing in present-day society, with an open eye to the future and further developments.

To address the question, particular attention needs to be given to areas where clinical or community nursing time is taken up not in essential nursing care but in administrative duties. Such duties appear to diminish the nurse's role and in many instances take nurses away form the work they are most qualified to undertake, that of direct patient care.

If a historical perspective is taken to form a base, the nurses of the pre-Miss Nightingale era were untrained, though hardworking, often

* Nursing is used to represent nursing, midwifery and health visiting.

in appalling conditions, and constantly at the bedsides of those in their care, in a semi-structured system following the Industrial Revolution and the breaking up of the large family unit. Medicine was in its infancy, and 'cured' very few ailments following what we would consider today to be barbaric methods of treatment. The development of training for nurses, primarily through Miss Nightingale's efforts, highlighted the role of bedside practitioners. The role remained constrained through both the type of entrant and through the then slow developments in medical treatments. As medical knowledge grew, so did the role of the nurse.

In historical terms, using a clock face to represent time, we could suggest that if an hour is used to represent the last three hundred years, the time taken in the development of the profession of nursing is no more than ten minutes, barely enough time to draw breath. It is suggested that it is the rapidity of development that has heightened nursing's 'coping' mechanisms. Such mechanisms have assured nursing's future to some degree, but they may also have pushed nurses into changes they were not ready for. In order to build the background to the technological developments, a few moments of reflection may now help to focus thoughts and establish questions within the remit of the original question of why nurses should concern themselves with computers.

It has often been said that in nursing today, nurses with most patient contact are the junior students in the general area and that the further up the hierarchical ladder they go the further away from the bedside they get. Is there a place for computers at the bedside, thus potentially increasing patient contact time for all concerned in their care? The amount of paperwork at ward level is staggering, and with continued changes in the overall structure of the Health Service the growth in administrative duties is not dwindling. Is it in this area that information technology (in the form of computers) can help? It should be stated at this point that information technology is a broader concept than that generally associated with the use of computers. Computers are analytical tools, with information technology as the gathering, processing and delivery of information data from a variety of sources.

In education too, there are increasing demands made upon the teaching staff in administrative areas, together with demands to know how individual students learn. In small groups this is feasible by traditional methods but when faced with larger groups as is occurring with schools amalgamating into colleges and the development and implementation of curricula for Project 2000, the learning styles of individuals can be lost whilst attempting to attain the required standard for all students. Would computers help in education?

A problem for all involved in the development of computer and information technology tools has, and always will be that of 'mechanization' versus 'computerization'. The concept is that mechanization is the transfer of manual practices to the computer, so that everything becomes faster and possibly outwardly more efficient, but the computer tool is used merely as a storage device working in exactly the same way as the manual system. A computerized system, by the very nature of the process capacity of the technological tool, demands that the developer considers the implications of current working practices and determines a way of harnessing the computer power to enhance those practices and integrate the flow of information for the benefit of the organization. Further discussion based upon the premise that the Health Service has mechanized rather than computerized is considered later.

ADMINISTRATIVE USES OF COMPUTERS

The present career structure in nursing is varied and yet constraining. There are many avenues through which to travel in order to find the one that best reflects the individual's needs. Often in following one path the original career plan is lost through 'tacking' within the system, until such time as the planned direction is transposed into another plan. Due to the salary structure it is necessary for some to climb rather than take sideways steps, but in climbing the administrative duties become greater. The amount of paperwork is sometimes overwhelming, but it is possible through harnessing technology in an effective manner that a reduction in both time and energy may be forthcoming. If this can be done, then individuals can have reflective space in order to develop in their role.

Take an example of a traditional method versus an assistive method utilizing the technology available in the role of Director of Nursing. Directors are responsible for the nursing staff within their domain. Traditionally, information regarding the staff is maintained in written format, requiring manual retrieval and updating. The retrieval aspect can be long and laborious, extremely time-consuming and frequently inaccurate in statistical information gleaned. The confidentiality aspect, too, can present difficulties, in that the information may be stored in filing cabinets into which access, even when the cabinets are locked, can be relatively easily gained. Alternatively the information may be stored in 'Kardex' form and thus even lower security is maintained on the information. Computers have a passion for numbers and statistics, and can be made accessible by password (or log-in code) only. Such a code uniquely identifies the user to the computer. The password can be assessed by the computer and only certain information can be retrieved depending upon the chosen policy of the Director. The information can be displayed or formatted to suit individual requirements, thus permitting ease of identification of required information and presentation of the information in an understandable form. Where such a system is in operation, the Director can maintain a complete picture of the staff at all times, ensuring that study-leave entitlement, preretirement courses, maternity leave, holidays, sickness, etc., are planned into the overall strategy for the forthcoming year. Similarly, the qualifications of staff could be ascertained quickly should an emergency arise. It is this type of information and the control of such information that a Director requires in order to steer the ship with confidence and autonomy.

CLINICAL USES OF COMPUTERS

In the clinical area, the often-heard cry is for more staff. The cries frequently go unanswered due to the lack of reliable relevant quantifiable data. It would be naive to imagine that lack of information was the only reason, but the others regarding manpower generally are outside the remit of this book.

One area of relevant data is that of estimating the dependencies/workload indices of the patients and then, through a recognized formula, determining the establishment requirements to match the dependency in order to assure a maintenance of appropriate standards in nursing care.

The traditional manual method employed to produce dependency/establishment estimates is slow, laborious and frequently out of date in a short space of time. Through the use of computerized nursing records (of which examples are given later in book), it is possible to have the data on an hourly basis, indicating fluctuations. In order for this to occur, during the design of the computer system information is fed into the computer that ensures accurate calculations to the required formula. As in any use of such systems, it is also part of the design process to enable production of the information in a clear and easily understood manner relevant to the request for information.

The sister (charge nurse) can then use the data in the argument for (or against) the need for staff. Similarly the person in charge can be in a position to plan the staggering of routine admissions with the medical staff in order to assure all concerned of the quality of care expected in that environment. Traditional methods of form completion rely heavily upon the nursing staff and reduces time with the patients. This too can easily be handled through the use of computers in the wards linked to the appropriate departments using easy entry of the information on a once-only basis.

There is a growing requirement to gather information and measure variance for performance indicators in the clinical area and for quantifiable data to assist with the measurement of the quality of care. The calculation and measurement of set indicator standards could be potential uses for computerization.

EDUCATIONAL USES OF COMPUTERS

In this area, statistical information on students' progress through their training was traditionally maintained by hand. Today there appears to be a ready acceptance of computerized systems to remove the drudgery of this task and to give the officer in charge more creative time in order to plan for changes.

Methods of teaching, based on 'chalk and talk' are effective in delivering information; the marking of essays, project work and multiple choice papers do assess the students' progress, but none of these directly assist in understanding the student. If designed appropriately, a computer learning package, in combination with more traditional approaches, can assist in determining the learning style of the student. Through a well-designed computer-assisted learning package the computer can follow the path of students as they go through the package, thus highlighting each student's area of competence and non-competence. (Such a measurable ability is not true of many computer learning packages; further discussion of this area takes place later in the book.)

Understanding by students of information technology can also be developed by permitting them access to some of the tools technology (the computer) offers; for example, by preparing project assignments using wordprocessing, analysing data using statistical tools, and arranging data suitable to their needs through spreadsheets or databases. Computers in education should not merely be seen as packages used for 'drill and practice' or remedial study.

WHERE TO NOW?

Through the use of the limited number of instances above, perhaps the question of why nurses should consider using information technology in the form of computers is beginning to be answered. Finding a total answer that solves all known problems of practice and organization is unlikely ever to occur, for as we find one solution through the use of computers and information technology another problem demanding further solution may appear, but we must feel secure in ourselves in order to find the computer solutions initially. We owe it to nursing to be aware of the technology and the power of information within an organization.

The following chapters should assist in attaining such security and base of knowledge. It is the development of nursing knowledge in the area of computers and information technology that underlies the purpose of this book.

NURSES' ACCEPTANCE OF NEW TECHNOLOGY

A new method of working is often not easily instigated and frequently the method and tool of delivery clouds the actual use to those most concerned. For example, in the introduction of the Nursing Process, the method and tool of delivery were clear enough in most instances, the paperwork being the tool, the method being the completing of the paperwork within the columns identified. Many appeared to believe that the Nursing Process was a model of nursing; yet it is a tool in itself, to which a nursing model can be assigned. Through being clouded by the 'paperwork' the main thrust of the Nursing Process, that of systematizing nursing care into a holistic and objective management structure, appears to have been lost. Are we taking the same approach to the introduction of computers and information technology and not seeing the wood for the trees?

We, as nurses, tend to be wary of change. There are many valid reasons for this, but there is a tendency to react negatively to new ideas rather than analysing the method and implication of them.

If, earlier, we answered positively to the question of why nurses should understand computers, and can see a use for computers, then why has it taken so long for us to harness the technology? There are a number of reasons for this, including:

1. lack of computer knowledge by nurses;
2. historically poor or non-relevant computer systems used;
3. fear of computers;
4. belief by nurses that computers would never reach the wards; and
5. reluctance to invest heavily in limited tested systems.

The list above could relate to other adult phobias by the removal of the link to computers and nurses and the insertion of, for example, swimming or driving. A few years ago due in part to the list above, technological changes were virtually ignored by nurses. There appeared to be two opposite technological extremes involved. At one end were the enthusiasts whose attitude tended towards uncritical acceptance of the benefits offered, and at the other end were those who wanted nothing whatsoever to do with the emerging technologies and did all in their power to dissuade others from attempting to tame the technological beast, with dread warnings of the awful consequences that would ensue.

It is apparent that nursing as a whole, did not fall into the category of uncritical enthusiasm but, to be honest, neither did it truly fall into the other extreme. A more likely explanation is that during the computer technology revolution's embryonic stage nurses hid their heads in the sand in the hope that computer technology would go away.

The late 1970s saw a new dawn. Nurses were more open to the computer technology that surrounded them in offices, shops and the home. The words 'computer', 'database' and 'information technology' became common in the English language and there was greater use of technology in hospital equipment for direct and non-direct patient care.

> '. . . a massive penetration of powerful computers into people's lives. That this will happen there can be no doubt. The calculator, the electronic game and the digital watch were brought to us by a technical revolution.'
>
> Papert, S. 1980

The technical revolution assisted in enhancing patient-monitoring equipment, laboratory equipment and administrative equipment, but did not encroach on nursing in any comprehensive way. The period 1979–83 saw attempts at developing computerized systems for use by the clinically-based nurse; it also saw rapid development in the use of computers in administrative areas of nursing, and the emergence of computer use in education.

The fuse had been lit. Part of the ignition process is thought to have been during Information Technology Year (1982) when an international conference was held in London, dedicated to the subject of computers in nursing. The conference heightened awareness of the uses to which computers could be harnessed, yet the main area of nursing-directed uptake appears not to have been in the clinical field but rather in the educational setting.

At the 1982 conference, Dr Barry Barber suggested in his paper *Computers Need Nursing* that,

> '. . . it (the computer) offers opportunities for providing something extra – extra information, extra insight, extra monitoring, extra control or extra time.'

Certainly the above would seem to be valid points, worth striving for in our present clinical, community and educational climate. Dr Barber did, however, continue by saying,

> 'Systems can be fast, powerful and incredibly useful if they have been properly designed. Clear objectives and purposeful analysis lead to useful systems.'

MECHANIZED OR COMPUTERIZED?

It is becoming increasingly evident that computer systems have been designed and implemented to meet short-term ill-defined goals. Computer systems have been saddled with the task of undertaking information storage mirroring those previously undertaken manually. There is limited retrieval of the stored information, but rarely sufficient to meet growing demands placed upon the computer system by the ever-growing information enquirers, such as various administrative of clinically-based departments.

In essence what has occurred can be simply explained. Computers have been implemented to continue the working practices of the staff who once completed the information manually, and little or no thought has been given to using the full power of the computer for information integration across various computer applications, or to addressing the larger and possibly more difficult area of assessing current working practices to ascertain if any positive alterations could be made. For example, prior to computerization, a number of the same forms containing the same information may have been required across departments; thus triplicate (or more) copies are made. Strange as it may seem, there are computer systems around today that continue this paper/form practice. However, had some thought been applied, there may well have been a way to remove the need for multiple forms and actually use the computer technology to transfer information between departments. Frequently occurrences can be found where there is obvious duplication of information, with no apparent way forward toward information interchange or computerization in its true form.

It is remarkably easy to develop a computer system to hold information, to mirror current practices and to deliver required information and obviously this has occurred throughout the Health Service, possibly at high cost. The hard part is to examine current working practices and determine the most effective way forward for all concerned, to permit computerized development with information not technology as the key, and to use technology merely as a vehicle to assist in information flow through a department, organization or across boundaries larger than imagined before. It is very easy to place a computer box on someone's desk with some sort of package housed within it. Expectations of immediate understanding seem to proliferate, particularly among managers, whereas it is much harder than this to develop a computer system to meet the needs of staff and the organization. Thus it is obvious why mechanization has frequently been selected as the way forward.

Computerize or mechanize; the decision must be yours. Suffice to say that the latter will ensure information is stored and is easy to examine. However, the former, computerization, will be the way forward for both the professions and the organization.

COMPUTERS – THE WAY FORWARD

Our responsibility to ourselves, to those in training and to those in our care is that we acquaint ourselves with a knowledge base in the technological arena in order that properly designed systems can work for us rather than us working for the systems (computers).

In a general clinical environment today, we experience a plethora of technology; intravenous infusion pumps, monitors, blood sugar estimators to name but a few. These have been accepted as lateral extensions to the clinical nurse's role. These 'tools' are viewed as aiding nurses rather than hindering them. Even so, it has been suggested that some nurses look at a monitor first and then at the patient, exhibiting, perhaps, a reliance on technology. Do we wish such a reliance to be paramount? This is a question containing much for nursing to consider.

We, as nurses, are trained to a high level in our profession, but should we now learn another aspect – that of making computers do what we want through writing programs ourselves? In no way is this believed to be the required step forward. We must know what computers are capable of doing, we must learn how to communicate with the professionals in the computer world, but a 'team' approach is the more favourable step to be taken, in order that the 'whole' can be taken into account.

'Nurses are becoming more aware of computer technology, are gaining confidence in using the enhanced information thus made available and learning to specify their requirements in relation to their objectives in providing patient care and planning the services of the future.'

'. . . nurses have been the innovators and driving force but have not hesitated to ask for and have received advice and help from specialist staff which has enabled them to achieve their objectives.'

Warne, B. E. M. 1983

It is possible that through the rapid growth of computer technology we have lost sight of our role as members of the 'team'. Many around us use jargon with which we are not acquainted, and rather than lose face we sometimes make assumptions based on incomplete knowledge and then wonder why our involvement is minimal at later stages. Unfortunately a comparison could be made with the Hans Christian Andersen fairy tale, *The Emperor and His Suit of Clothes*, where the

Emperor accepted the words of others rather than believing his own eyes.

As Warne suggests, we are the innovators, but we do need others to ensure that effective translation of our ideas occurs. These 'translators' should be viewed not as directing us but rather as assisting us to meet our demands and needs, just as we meet those of the patients in our care.

As the subject of the book is the use of computers, there is obvious emphasis upon the fact that computers can help in our environment. It should be stated that this is not always the case, and there are many examples where the implementation of computer systems has caused great distress and anguish. Generally the reason for lack of successful use has been due to the poor design of the system and a lack of involvement by those at the 'sharp end' of using it.

Sufficient training has also frequently been lacking together with poor evaluation of the system's suitability to perform the task required. The following chapters should assist in giving a knowledge base to nurses, and each section answers questions previously raised to the author concerning different computers, including demystification of the jargon, use of prepared packages or designing individual requirements for both nursing and education of nurses. In conclusion, the future of the technology and how it can help nursing and other health care professionals in the management of those in their care are considered.

We do not all have to become computer enthusiasts; indeed it is good to have sceptics available to discuss development practicalities. However, it has been suggested (James, 1991) that there is a continuum present; at the one extreme the 'doers' who love to sit at a computer terminal all day and frequently speak in a language unknown to most of us; at the other end the 'thinkers' who accept, to a point, that computer technology is valuable and are aware of its potential, but do not feel a need to tap away at a computer keyboard. It is necessary for nursing to have a mixture of 'doers' and 'thinkers' in order to progress. It is fitting that each of us should determine where on the continuum we are most comfortable, for we must sit somewhere upon the continuum and not bury our heads in the sand like ostrichs and expect computers and information technology to go away. Berg, at the 1982 conference (The Impact of Computers on Nursing) made a statement that might be worth considering before moving on. Read it in the light of administrative pressure towards the use of computers and ask yourselves on which side of the choice spectrum you would rather fall in order to maintain control of the nursing environment.

'The choice is there and the time to make the choice is now. The decision must be whether to act traditionally and have change thrust upon the profession from the outside or to anticipate this revolution in nursing practice, familiarize nurses with it, and prepare them to take an active part in the introduction of computers in the nursing community . . . so that computer technology is used to assist nurses in improving the quality of nursing practice and thus the quality of patient care.'

Berg, C. M. 1983

Chapter Two

The development of the computer

In this chapter, examination will be made of the differences and similarities between the computers which are available to meet the various needs of nurses and nursing. The contents of this and the remaining chapters may also help the reader in discerning the differences between computerization and mechanization. A list of computer terms which may be unfamiliar to the reader is given in Appendix A at the back of the book.

A computer is nothing by itself; thus brief explanations will be given of some of the additional pieces of equipment regularly found attached to computers. As mentioned in the previous chapter, the word 'computer' is not synonymous with the phrase 'information technology', although this is frequently assumed. It is always pertinent to assemble the information before deciding on the tools (whether technological or non-technological) we require.

One of the first considerations therefore is to determine what is meant by 'information technology'. The term is frequently used, but is it appropriate in many instances? To break down the phrase, the first element of 'information' can be defined as

'Informing, telling; thing told, knowledge, (desired) items of knowledge; news.'

Concise Oxford Dictionary

The understanding of the word is unlikely to be incorrectly assumed in most cases. The second element, that of 'technology', is sometimes more difficult. A dictionary definition is

'(Science of) practical or industrial art(s); application of science.'

Concise Oxford Dictionary

This, perhaps, poses more difficulty in understanding and general use. It would appear that the 'application of science' aspect is the one that has led to the almost immediate assumption that 'technology' has to do with developments in machinery, be that computers or cars.

In conversation, the term 'technology' can refer to developments in medicine, physics, chemistry and other more human-associated fields. It is in the joining of the two words that a term is formed which is generally recognized to mean mechanical processing of knowledge (information). The computer plays a vital role as the 'mechanical' element of the equation, but is by no means the whole equation.

The term 'information technology' is a relative newcomer to our language and possibly reflects the importance we place upon the use of mechanical tools to assist in knowledge gathering, processing and delivery. It must not be forgotten, however, that the vital element in the whole arena of information technology is the human element.

From the brief discussion above, it is perhaps recognized that there is a dilemma as to whether to commence with a review of the machinery available to us, or with a description of what information requirements we have and then to find a machine and application software to meet those requirements. In many instances in our health care use of information technology, the latter course is not possible, as decision-making frequently occurs away from the effective domain for which the machinery is intended.

If you are faced with a computer, it may be pertinent to commence with the technology, but please note that this may not always be the most effective approach. The discussion that follows is based upon the premise that when 'technology' is used it refers to computers and thus in this instance consideration will only be given to historical and present developments involving machines now called computers.

A sobering thought in today's fast-moving world is that the first recognized computer was designed in 1833 by Sir Charles Babbage. His machine, full of valves and motors, was called the 'Analytic Engine'; quite an appropriate name when one considers the functioning of the machine, and the use of the word 'engine' is understandable as this was the only word available in the language at the time. Babbage's 'engine' was capable of working out simple numerical problems, but the time taken was frequently longer than it would have taken to do them mentally. The astounding fact was that it was capable of working out the problem in the first place.

It was over a hundred years before the next major step forward in the use of machines to work out problems for humans was made, and this time the machine was used to decode messages sent during the Second World War. The machine was called 'Colossus I'. Certainly it lived up to its name, because it was huge and took a great deal of tender loving care to ensure that it continued working in the manner for which it was designed.

Following the breakthrough Colossus I afforded, the development of computers has been extremely rapid; there are now hand-held machines available with capabilities far in excess of Colossus. When the word 'computer' began to be recognized, as a term for a machine that could solve mathematical problems (derived from the earlier word 'compute' meaning to determine logically mathematical solutions from given formulae), the development of machines began in earnest. As stated earlier the computer is capable of processing information; thus each machine of whatever size has a central processing unit (CPU). As a rule of thumb it used to be possible to determine the computer type by the size of the central processing unit. However, with current developments this is not always the only indicator of computer ability.

COMPUTERS

Historically, the first generally available computer was the mainframe (Figure 2.1). As with Colossus, it tended to be large and filled with

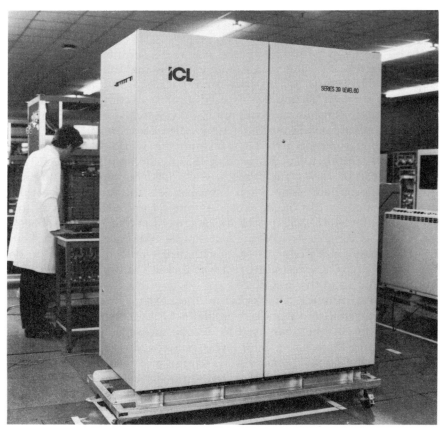

Figure 2.1 Part of a mainframe computer.

electrical gadgetry, requiring specially adapted rooms and a team of support staff. As the 'moving parts' inside computers were reduced so did the number of support staff, but the housing required has basically remained unchanged.

The CPU for such a machine has many input and output devices serving the central processing elements. The CPU itself is capable of millions of calculations per second and the attendant devices ensure that it is immediately able to call up the information it requires and produce, in human-readable format, the resulting information on screen or paper printout. Such large systems are in operation where a large amount of information processing is required and where there may be many users wishing to gain access to information at the same time, for example in banks, building societies and the police.

As production of non-moving 'hi-tech' parts progressed, so a reduction in the size of computers followed. The next group of computers to arrive were the minicomputers, tending to be smaller in size but having equal, or nowadays greater, capacity in their ability to process information quickly and to have many users connected to the system at the same time. Today the capacity differences between the mainframe and minicomputers are increasingly blurred. There appears to be more growth in the use of minicomputers, due possibly to the increased processing ability of minicomputers and their reduced need for specialist housing and attention. Such physical size differences can be seen in Figure 2.2.

In both figures the serving elements are still in evidence, the only recognizable difference being in the size of the main processing 'box', which ranges from that of two four-drawer filing cabinets to that of a single two-drawer filing cabinet.

The user feeds information into the computer through a terminal (the same for the mainframe and mini) and the terminal is usually connected by special cables to the CPU. There are two main types of terminal, either a visual display unit with keyboard (much like a typewriter) (Figure 2.3) or a keyboard alone. Sometimes the input can be through the use of cards, but frequently this does not allow for any immediate output to the user. The terminal does not have to be in the vicinity of the CPU; it can be in the same building or many miles away. Indeed there are satellite connections available today that allow for intercontinental communication with the CPU or for communication between differently sited terminals through the computer.

The next major breakthrough was the development of the microcomputer in the 1970s. This tended to be in the form of a 'workstation', where the CPU is housed in the same 'box' as that attached to the keyboard (Figure 2.4). Again, with developments in the storage capacity of the 'chip' these machines are now capable of processing vast amounts

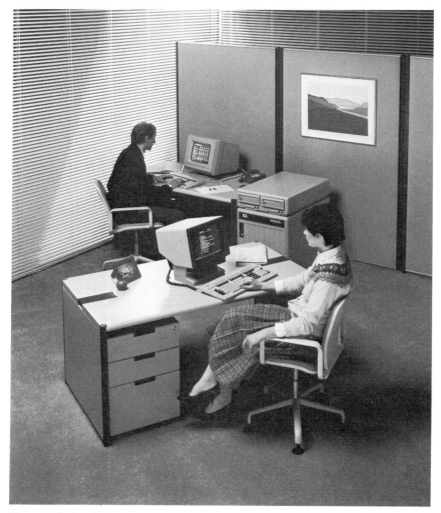

Figure 2.2 A minicomputer.

of data in a short space of time. Again the differences are blurred between some modern micro and older minicomputers through the development of microchip technology.

A chip is a silicon wafer and each layer of the wafer adds to the capacity of the chip. It has no moving parts and thus, once successfully manufactured, it should not falter in its tasks. The microcomputer has

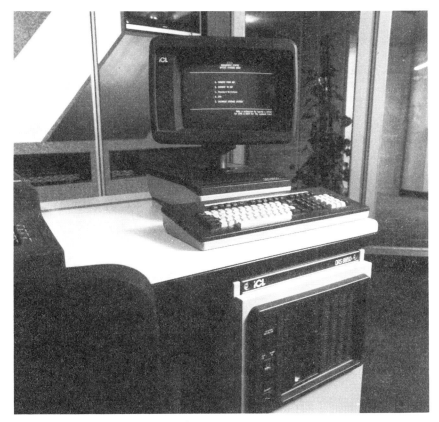

Figure 2.3 A computer terminal.

led to a greater use of computers through the lowering of prices and the fact that it requires very little in the way of support and maintenance from professionally trained staff. The microcomputer features all the elements of the other broad categories mentioned, its advantage being its portability and availability to the general public.

There is a general view that microcomputers can be further divided into two main categories; those for commercial and administrative duties (personal computers or PCs) and those for home use. The former tend to have larger memory and function capacities, using a wide selection of packages; the latter tend to be used exclusively for a required task, for example wordprocessing or games, although increasingly, due to reduction in price and increased availability, PCs are being used for home administration. The cost range of computers is as wide as the types available, from around £1 million for a large main-

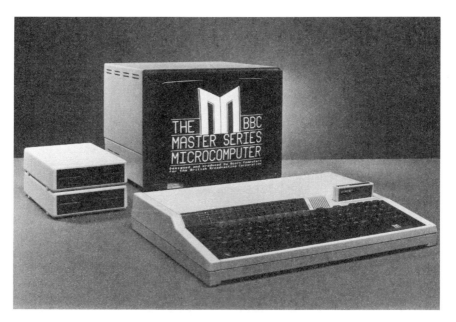

Figure 2.4 A microcomputer.

frame system, to under £100 for some microcomputers; hence the growth in microcomputer use by private users and organizations.

There are 'service' devices attached to microcomputers, which once again have been designed to require little attention, such as data storage on floppy discs which can be delivered through a normal mailing system, instead of the larger hard discs used by mainframes and minis which require special handling.

The microcomputer is capable of being connected with others of its kind and indeed with its larger 'brothers' through normal telephone lines and satellite links. Many organizations today look to microcomputers as the first choice, then link them together through a cabled network or to a larger CPU as their information needs grow.

Development of the microcomputer has facilitated the use of computers in our schools and homes. Some people now argue that it should be every person's right in this country to have access to computers, in order that an understanding of information technology is available to all.

With the advances in computer technology, the size of the computer has reduced further. Now on the market are hand-held and lap-top computers which are capable of storing large amounts of data and retrieving it whenever the user wishes: in a client's home, in the car, on the train, and many other places. Again such developments give greater flexibility and freedom in the use of computers.

'SERVICE' DEVICES

In order to explain some of the points above, it was necessary to use terms that may not be familiar. The next section will, it is hoped, clarify the terms and their relationship with the main computer. As with any knowledge retrieval and processing, such as using a book, there has to be storage of initial information. This is known as data storage and, for computers, tends to come in five basic formats as follows:

1. cassette
2. tape (reel to reel)
3. floppy disc
4. hard disc
5. chip.

Each of these either stores information in a coded form or in 'files' where a complete section is stored for retrieval, just as we might keep a variety of files in a cabinet under different subject headings.

Cassette

We are all used to storing musical material on this medium, which can also be used to store conversations or monologues in natural human language. In the early days of microcomputers all computer data was stored in such a fashion, when the computer would select the start point, play the section required and 'read in' the data. If requested, the computer would transfer data from the CPU to the cassette for retrieval later.

The difficulties with cassette tape are essentially twofold, the first being that it is slow in both retrieval and storage of data, the second that cassette tape has a tendency to stretch with prolonged use, thus causing some data to be lost or irretrievable, in that the computer can no longer find the right point at which to start or finish, or indeed find the data required.

Cassette data storage certainly fulfilled a valuable function at a time when there was nothing else available and through the use of such a storage medium many lessons have been learnt. Some microcomputers still use a modified version of the cassette tape, such as Sinclair's 'micro drive tapes', which were specially designed to reduce difficulty in tape stretch. Those with such storage devices find them quite satisfactory.

This form of storage is not used with mainframe or minicomputers for primary data storage, but is used by some as a secondary 'back-up' data store.

Tape (reel to reel)

This storage medium is used with mainframe and minicomputers generally as back-up data storage. The tape is specialized, as is the machinery upon which it is used. Due to the specialization, the retrieval can be very fast. The recorded tape is transportable as long as certain precautions are taken. These precautions include avoiding X-ray equipment, such as security systems at airports. There is still the difficulty of tape stretch, although this is reduced through specialization and specific use.

Floppy disc

This storage medium is generally used with microcomputers. The floppy discs superficially resemble musical discs of the 45 r.p.m. variety, and there are several sizes other than the common 5¼ inch, both smaller and larger. The general movement is towards 3½ inch disks enclosed within a hard protective case, suitable for carrying in a jacket pocket or handbag. The medium remains magnetic, as with the cassette tape, and data is read through specially adapted drives. The main advantages are that the discs are capable of speedy retrieval and storage and large amounts of data can be stored. Discs are easily transportable and easily stored.

The capacity of the disc depends mainly upon two factors; the first being the type of content material used, the second being its formatting. When you obtain an unused disc, it has no information contained on it. Prior to saving information from the computer you must format the disc. The format process prepares the disc into sections into which data for storage can be filed, rather like a new drawer in a filing cabinet. Before using the drawer, file dividers must be inserted into which the files are then placed; if the dividers were not in place the drawer would not be easily accessed as all the files would be piled up in the drawer. Generally, in computer terms, the format is either 40 or 80 track (high density), 720Kb or 1.44Mb (high density), with the 80 track/1.44Mb version giving greater potential storage facilities.

Once a disc has been formatted for one particular make of computer it will not work on another. For example, a disc formatted using an IBM PC will not work on an Acorn BBC microcomputer (unless you are using an emulator package and probably through RISC technology) and vice versa. If a disc formatted on an IBM PC is used with a microcomputer of a different make which is 100% IBM compatible it should function normally.

The disc can be damaged (corrupted) through mishandling, but if the exterior packaging instructions are followed this reduces the possibility of damage. Floppy discs should not be placed near electrical charges, for example on the floor of London underground trains as an electrical discharge from the train may corrupt the disc. Generally, magnetic fields such as airport baggage check-ins are safe, but it is accepted that you may wish to hand discs to the security personnel rather than carry them through the body scanner.

Hard disc

As the name suggests, these discs are not flexible; they come in a variety of sizes and a variety of storage capabilities. Some are single, with information on both sides, some are in banks of discs.

These discs require a different type of drive from the floppy disc, but the basic function is the same, that of using a magnetic head to 'read' and 'imprint' data on to the storage medium. A hard disc is generally used to store very large amounts of information and may be housed either inside or outside the CPU cabinet. In many PCs there is a hard disc housed in the main casing of the computer which tends to range between 20Mb and 50Mb. Hard discs tend to present greater problems with transportation than any of the above, since internal hard discs must be 'parked' or 'dismounted' prior to moving the computer or when use is no longer required, for example at the end of the day, in order to protect the disc and the magnetic head. Some modern computers do this automatically.

Chip

The silicon microchip has enhanced all the above forms of storage. Suffice it to say that the chip stores information in a very different way from the magnetic medium. The chip has no moving parts visible to the naked eye, but the design implements metal gates or switches to open and close allowing information to be stored or retrieved, as seen in Figure 2.5.

There are two broad categories of chips generally available: Read Only Memory (ROM), and Random Access Memory (RAM). With the ROM, the chip acts as a retrieval element only. When data has been stored on the chip the user can call up that information but cannot add to the information on the chip for later use. This form is generally used for commercially produced software or courseware. RAM allows additional data storage in the machine to which it is attached (generally

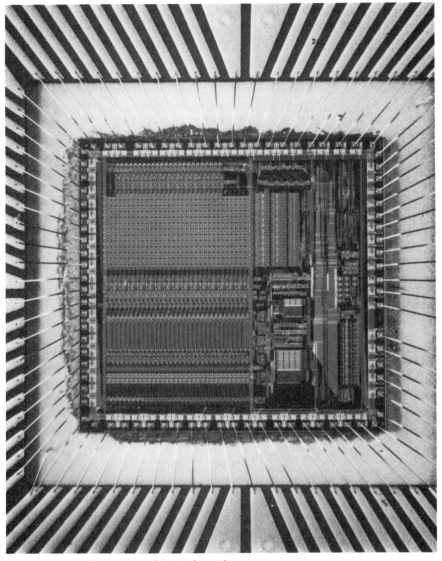

Figure 2.5 A silicon microchip (enlarged).

a microcomputer); hence the user can 'communicate' with the chip and add data for retrieval later. The RAM size of a microcomputer (or PC) is often referred to as the 'working space' within the computer.

Other important devices for communication with the central processing unit are:

1. visual display unit (VDU)
2. keyboard
3. printer
4. mouse (and other graphic devices)
5. telephone connections.

The computer is a dumb machine; it cannot act instinctively, but must be told exactly its course of action, hence the necessity for the user to be able to communicate with the internal mechanism. The devices for doing this are generally called 'input' and 'output' devices: under input comes the keyboard and mouse; under output are the VDU and printer. The following descriptions are merely of the hardware (the items that can be touched). The communication with the computer in order to make it behave as we would wish (software) is covered in the next chapter.

Visual display unit (VDU)

In many respects this resembles a television screen, which can be either, mono (one screen colour and one print colour) or full colour. The VDU displays both the user's input and the computer's output in most instances, which may be in the form of text, graphics or programming data. Advances in technology have not escaped the VDU, where the major step forward is the use of 'touch screens'. Here the user points either with a finger or a light pen touching the screen, and the user's choice is communicated to the CPU, thus allowing for fast and simple information retrieval and storage. In the past, the VDU was unable to show anything other than that directly related to the computer. With the advent of video interacting with computer programs, developments have ensured that a video picture can be simultaneously displayed on the VDU with computer instructions.

Keyboard

In most instances this resembles the traditionally accepted QWERTY keyboard such as that on a typewriter, but additional items are a full numeric keypad and special function keys. The keyboard is either an integrated part of the main body of the computer or attached separately to permit ease in positioning. Some keyboards are specially adapted to meet the needs of specific groups of users, for example children (Figure 2.6), or for computers dedicated to a single application.

The keyboard is generally the main method of communication with the CPU for input purposes. There are developments in voice activation but these are not yet generally available.

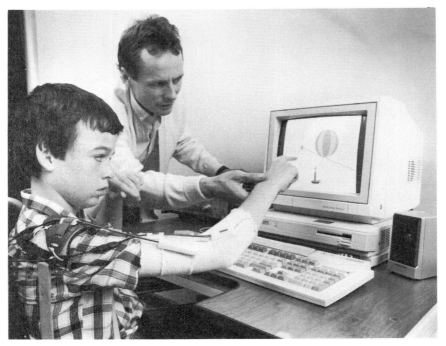

Figure 2.6 Child using specially adapted keyboard.

Printer

Alongside the VDU, the printer is the main output device for information. There are two main methods in which printers work, either by impacting the character onto the paper a line at a time, or by preparing a whole page before it is printed. The first method, impact printing, includes daisywheel and dot matrix printers; the second method, page printers, includes laser, ink jet and bubble jet printers. Consideration here will be given to the daisywheel, dot matrix and laser printers. The daisywheel uses a 'wheel' of characters and the result cannot be distinguished from a normal typewriter; thus this type of printer is used for producing high-quality letters and documents. There is very limited ability to produce graphical representation with these printers other than very basic block graphs. Daisywheel printers have a tendency to be noisy and reasonably slow in comparison with the other types of printer. The noise is generated through the character being hit against a ribbon on to the paper. It is possible to have different print types, for example italic or courier, by inserting different daisywheels.

The dot matrix group of printers tend to be quieter and faster. The method of character printing is either through a series of ink dots being spurted on to the paper, or dots passed through a ribbon. The quality of print varies. The lower the number of 'dots' the lower the quality of printout. Generally nine 'pins' (or dots) give the lowest quality and the pins are arranged in three columns of three dots (matrix). The highest quality printer in common use has 24 pins arranged in four columns of six dots. Due to demand, most high-pin dot matrix printers tend to be near letter quality (NLQ) as in the daisywheel, but generally it is possible to distinguish between a normal typewriter and a dot matrix printer. It is possible to produce graphics with most of these printers and some of them offer a colour facility. Different print types are possible, but unlike the daisywheel, these are generally selected through the computer program application rather than through altering or adapting the printer itself. Included in this group of printers are those called 'plotters' which are dedicated to producing graphics as their major function, although some use coloured pens. Again colour is possible.

A new development is the laser printer, where the characters or graphics are carbonized on to the paper. The printer initially receives information from the computer, then decifers this to produce areas on the paper where the black carbon will be used to form characters or graphics. These printers tend to handle single sheets of paper only. There are two main types, Postscript and non-Postscript. The name 'Postscript' refers to a particular software package, where the printer ensures a high definition of graphics and text. The laser printer is reasonably fast and very efficient in its production of 'hard copy' material. As the cost of Postscript laser printers is still very high, this group of printers is generally found only where there is adequate reason for its use. There are inexpensive non-Postscript laser printers now available, giving a good resolution output, resulting in an increase in their use.

Mouse

This is an input device, (as illustrated in Figure 2.7), and its development has been due to user demands for something other than a keyboard to input information but cheaper to install than touch screens. The resulting increase in the use of 'windows' and 'icons' can largely be traced back to the mouse. The mouse is used to direct single commands to the computer. It either sits on a special mat or can be used on a desk top beside the computer, and is used mainly with microcomputers.

The mouse, which is attached by a lead to the computer, has one or more 'keys' and fits neatly into the hand. A roller ball on the underside sends movement signals to the CPU. The movement of the mouse is

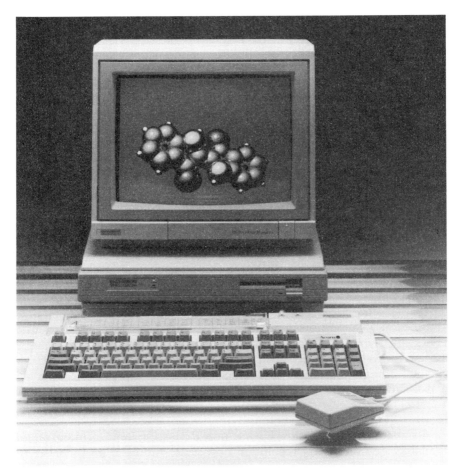

Figure 2.7 Microcomputer comprising VDU, keyboard and three-button mouse.

displayed on the screen. The key or keys are pressed when a selection is to be made. For example, on a three-key mouse the keys may correspond to 'execute', 'menu' or 'cancel'.

The use of such devices allows for computer use without any typing skills, and also permits the drawing of pictures, plans or other graphics without the user needing any special programming skills. In some earlier machines the full package included a ROM chip that was inserted into the computer to 'drive' the mouse functions as an additional feature to the original computer.

Telephone connections

A vast world is opened to the computer user through telephone connections. In the past mainframe computers were attached to users through specially adapted wires, some of which travelled many thousands of miles. Now already installed telephone lines without any adaptation are used.

To facilitate the telephone connection of micro, mini and mainframe computers there are a number of items used. The first is a ROM chip or disk package to 'drive' the terminal element of the computer (communications software), thus making the computer behave as a terminal for a variety of data sources. This tends to be 'menu-driven' for ease of use. Secondly, the public telephone system is used, through a normal line, even one attached to a switchboard. Thirdly, to convert the computer signals into those compatible with telephone signals, a modem is used.

The public telephone system is designed to carry analogue signals but the computer operates on digital signals so a series of conversions must take place.

COMPUTER → MODEM → TELEPHONE → MODEM → COMPUTER
digital   convert   analogue   convert   digital

The name 'modem' is derived from the work the box does. The initial conversion of digital to analogue is called 'modulation', the second conversion of analogue back to digital is called 'demodulation'; hence a MODEM MOdulates and DEModulates signals.

With such a massive communication system available there have been many changes in the way in which we view work and the workplace. For example, it no longer becomes necessary to be based in a particular area in the country, and working from home with a link to the main office is possible. Rather than reducing levels of communication there is an enormous increase in communication networking for information storage, processing and retrieval. Indeed, through the development of car telephones, it is now possible to use computer communication in a car fitted with the required equipment.

Banks use technological network communication to transfer information between branches and head offices, and when you use a bank service or switch card, your balance is checked via such a link. It is now possible, with satellite communication, to check your bank balance whilst in a foreign country, the whole communication taking approximately ten seconds. Other functions for which such a network can be used include letter communication between individuals or groups, transference of files to a central source or to identified individuals, computer connections rather than telephone connections for conferences, interrogation of computer databases, and even shopping or checking on train schedules from home.

The scene in the generation of technological tools to aid daily living is anything but static, and the examples given above are but a few of the more likely service devices that will be encountered. Chapter 6 gives a hint of what is to come. In the next chapter, consideration will be given to the software (programs) and the uses of the items mentioned above. It will be shown that the computer in all its forms works for the user, and should not be regarded as something to be afraid of or to be avoided.

Chapter Three

The systematic approach to design

'The Centipede was happy quite
Until the toad in fun said,
'Pray which leg comes after which?'
This wrought her mind to such a pitch
She lay distracted in a ditch
Considering how to run.'
                    Anonymous; Seymour Papert, 1980

As stated in the last chapter, the dilemma is again which element to tackle first with regard to the hardware/software debate. The short poem above possibly demonstrates the problem, the point being that in our role we understand needs and problems and can usually find solutions. However, when faced with a more regimented systematic approach such as designing a system suitable for use with computers, our reaction may not be so clearly defined. Indeed, we may have to look more carefully into the problem than we first thought, and such examination is vital to the successful use of computers. Analysis is the key to successful design.

A common example is that of building a cupboard at home, or tackling a new untried recipe, both large and relatively complicated tasks, which may appear daunting – rather like the problem of the centipede. If the task is taken in logical stages, fears may be reduced. Initially the need for such a cupboard or new recipe is considered, we might ask whether alternative arrangements could be made within the present storage capacity of the home, or whether we could consider repeating a previous recipe. If neither is viable, then the second stage commences; the type of storage or people for whom the recipe is intended will determine into which room the cupboard must go or the basic ingredients of the recipe. For the cupboard its position will be taken into account with size and capacity as other variables. The actual design will depend upon all the above factors, but another consideration will be whether this cupboard can be bought as a pack from a store (assessment may be made through visiting a number of stores) or whether you can build it yourself from scratch. The latter option brings many other questions to mind, such as 'Have I the tools?' 'Am I competent to build such a cupboard?' 'Do I have the time?' and 'What sort of materials do I need?' Similar considerations need to be given to the recipe. Indeed upon reflection it may be clear that a similar process is undertaken whenever you are tackling something new. As you can see, analysis is the major element, but if you spend time deciding prior to purchase of the goods, then there is less risk involved in actually building the cupboard or trying a new recipe. This analytical stage I call 'systems thinking'.

Before launching into considerations of systems thinking in relation to the use of computers, a little more knowledge needs to be assembled. The first part of this chapter will examine the non-hardware elements of computers and computing. Many books have been written in this area; thus the remit here is to give sufficient information for books to be read without confusion and misinterpretation. The second section of the chapter is concerned with analysis of need in order that suitability of computer application can be forthcoming.

A computer is not capable of anything unless it is commanded to do something, and the 'commanding' is where software comes in. The software is the way we communicate (on one level) with a computer; the intangible element made tangible by its connection with a computer and by the person sitting at the keyboard 'communicating' with the computer. Other words to mean software include:

1. program (American spelling)
2. package
3. courseware
4. applications software.

Through the use of these different terms it sometimes becomes difficult to comprehend what is being said. It is important that we realize that these words are interchangeable. In order to communicate we use language in two main forms, the spoken word and the written word. In this instance the use of non-verbal language is not relevant, for (fortunately) a computer cannot watch such signals from us, even at points of triumph and success. The building up of our own individual language has taken many years, through both informal and formal learning, and each of us holds a large vocabulary of words to use and, possibly more importantly, the knowledge of the appropriate context for using the words in order to make sense to the listener.

In specialist fields, words are added that include us in that specialist area, a sort of shorthand. Some argue that using an intimate or 'jargon' language prevents the inclusion of others, a fact that may well be true. In nursing, jargon is frequently found and in most instances it can be understood, but it could lead to misconceptions in other cases, especially through the use of abbreviations.

Computing too has a varied jargon, for to communicate with a computer we have to use a keyboard rather than the spoken word. We must use language that the computer comprehends; otherwise our efforts will be fruitless, leading to frustration in the use of a powerful information tool. Frustration can also be felt in any circumstances where our inclusion is not permitted through the use of specialized jargon, for instance, when a plumber is explaining the inner functionings of a central heating system.

If we examine more closely our method of communication with computers, it falls broadly into two main areas.

1. **Direct communication**. In the early days of computing, the major area of use was in the sciences, particularly mathematics and physics, and this still continues today. The link with mathematics led to worries from those without leanings in that direction as the languages used to communicate were alien to known spoken or written language. Such a language was 'octal,' which used figures with everything to the power of eight. However, these languages were close to the computer's own language, known as 'binary', where everything related to either '0' or '1', 'on' or 'off'. Those languages close to the computer's own communication understanding are termed 'low-level' languages and require little translation within the computer, thus taking up little room when used to make the computer work.

The 'high-level' languages are those that resemble our own spoken or written word. For example, assuming that we speak English, the learning of French may take some time, for we have to make a connection between what we know (English word or phrase) and what we don't know (French word or phrase). In the same way, the computer only knows binary and has to make a connection inside its own central processing unit to permit the use of a 'foreign' language; the bigger the translation the higher the level of language.

The use of a low-level or high-level language frequently depends upon the application required when using a computer, and this will be covered later.

2. **Indirect communication**. Here, rather than developing material from scratch, that is, the creation of software, we may use material already written. In this way we are indirectly communicating with the computer through the use of already prepared programs or courseware.

It is possible that most of us will communicate indirectly with computers either knowingly or unknowingly. For instance, every time we use an automatic cash dispenser outside a bank we communicate with a central computer; when filling a car tank with fuel we communicate to the cash desk through a computer. Indeed most of our day-to-day communication is controlled by computers.

In using a computer, that is, sitting in front of a keyboard, visual display unit and other peripherals, we would generally be using prepared packages. Most software now on the market has been evaluated and tends to be 'user-friendly', in that it assists the novice by telling them which 'buttons' to press at the right time. The user is led through the program and in most instances has very little say in the boundaries of the prepared program.

The knowledge required is generally only that of being able to turn the computer and peripherals on, ensuring that the storage medium (most commonly a disk) is correctly utilized and then working through the material that appears on the screen. In some instances, a working knowledge of using a keyboard (typewriter) may also be advantageous, if only in reducing time in hunting for the right key.

USER SOFTWARE

The market place for computers and computing is now producing more and more software for use by novices or those who want a result when using computers but do not wish to be bogged down in the in-depth knowledge required for intimate computer communication. The end user, or everyday non-computer person, has forced the computer companies into satisfying their need which has resulted in the growing delivery of packages that are said to be 'content-free' or 'content-flexible'. Concentration on these areas is considered in the following chapter.

It is interesting to note the swing that has occurred, away from computers being tools for an elite group requiring specially developed skills, to being tools for all with the direction coming from the end user rather than a computer 'expert'. We have developed our own specialist skills, and these must be valued both by ourselves and others in the working environment. Thus when considering computers any emphasis must come from the basis of knowledge and skills already attained. The growth in the computing area is promising as far as our use is concerned. It is no longer necessary to be able to program a computer in order to ensure that your requirements are met. Indeed as long as the logical system or content framework is known, the transference to computer is the easiest section, as with building the cupboard or trying out a new recipe. The 'technocrat' aspect has been reduced except in extremely specialized areas, enabling non-computing personnel to develop software pertinent to themselves. All that is required is the paper system and plenty of vision, although of course a commitment to the development underpins the entire concept.

PRACTICAL PLANNING FOR SOFTWARE

It all sounds easy, but there are barriers to forward momentum, and these barriers do tend to be placed inappropriately at times. By that I mean that rather than facing a problem and developing a solution we dismiss the problem as someone else's. Thus the barrier is formed indirectly as we perceive it, even though this barrier really is of our own doing. Another factor 'learnt' over recent years during times of crisis, is that of feeling unable to do anything, leading to apathy where nothing visionary is possible (laying 'distracted in a ditch . . .').

Some of the 'blocking' factors are due to a perceived dichotomy between systems of organization and planning. Our role, and quite rightly, is to care twenty-four hours a day for those in our wards, clinics, departments and community. We have all developed systems with our colleagues for dealing with people in our care. What frequently occurs are inaccurate assumptions following incomplete knowledge of other working practices (systems) involved in the team approach to care, which lead to misconceptions on all sides.

When our own system is questioned, the most common response is a belief that the questioner has no understanding of our role and frequently a stalemate occurs or, worse, our argument is dismissed as it appears to be on purely emotional grounds. Could it be that our own system is unclearly defined, hence the difficulty, on occasion, of being able to justify our actions? Have we considered our actions in the light of the larger organizational plan? Are others clear in their own role and function?

Prior to developing a computer system, we must be clear about our own system, determining what information is required by us and others in order to reduce overlap and misconceptions. Communication is of paramount importance to any change process. It must not be forgotten that everyone needs to be consulted prior to each stage and to be informed of progress during the development, for success rests upon all those involved feeling part of the change.

There are essentially six stages that are involved in completing the successful implementation of a system. In this instance the system is one that will involve the development of a learning package, but the same practices are true of any planning for change, including the change to a clinical computer system. It is always important to note that the formation of a 'team approach' will potentially produce better results in possibly a shorter space of time, so that all members of the team must have a full understanding of the end goal, and assumptions must not be made.

The six stages are:

1. knowledge of a need to change the present system;
2. concept of a new system or idea;
3. analysis of the present system;
4. design requirements of the new system;
5. implementation of the new system; and
6. evaluation of the change.

Knowledge of a need to change the present system

This is perhaps the most important stage, for until this decision is taken there is very little point in moving on to the other stages. It is not sufficient to 'feel' that something requires change; you must be committed to a change process based upon factual evidence.

In order to develop the factual evidence, you must examine the present system objectively, for it may be discovered upon thorough examination, that the present practice is satisfactory. Objective examination involves taking 'time out' from the general subjective stance. In some cases it may be necessary to involve people not directly associated with your system, and part of the process would be in having to explain your system to someone in the profession who is a total stranger.

Concept of the new system

If, after reflection, change is required you must have some embryonic idea of the new system in order to have a goal to work towards. Stories have often been cited of new designs being initially developed on the backs of envelopes, and indeed many a practical solution to a problem has been solved in this way. The point of an idea is that it forms a guideline, for at this stage it would be extremely unlikely that the full new system could be conceived. Do not try to be too definite at this stage, but do have a goal towards which you can aim.

The concept considers the whole, and the parts are to some extent irrelevant, but of course they will become important when you are in a later stage of planning as they will state the short- and possibly even the medium-term goals that go to build the greater whole.

Analysis of the present system

In reaching this stage, you are now convinced that there is a need for change and you have an idea of the new system, but you are like the centipede and need a starting point. This is it.

As with the DIY cupboard earlier, it is necessary to reflect upon your competence in relation to your requirement. Four essential questions must be asked during this reflection:

1. what?
2. where?
3. who?
4. how?

What needs to be changed? Is it, for example, a whole section of the curriculum to permit more flexible learning patterns, or just a small part of the curriculum, one 'lesson' area? Where does the change need to take place? Is it within your own 'system' or outside it? If in your own, does the development of a learning package mean, for example, a complete redesign of that section of the curriculum or of only a small part in order to satisfy a growing need?

To follow this theme a little further, and linking it with the next part, do not use something for the sake of it, or because someone is trying to persuade you. Do not accept the idea just to satisfy someone else. Be convinced yourself. Perhaps the greatest example of this was given in the fairy tale of the Emperor and his suit of clothes! To take a more every-day situation, have you bought something from someone just to get them off your doorstep, only to wonder later what you are going to do with your new acquisition?

The 'who?' element is an important one, not only in terms of the change and change agent but in terms of where you are directing the material and in terms of others within the total organization. Even a seemingly small change can send ripples through an organization, and they have a habit of turning into raging torrents if not addressed at an early stage. Involvement through communication with identified personnel is vital and should be carried out at all stages of development, from conception to evaluation. It is also strategically helpful to obtain commitment to the idea from senior personnel, thus adding weight to the idea and ensuring assistance in times of potential implementation crises.

The change agent is a key figure. With the learning package analogy, the agent of change may be the person who comes up with the idea and manages the change process, possibly through persuading a more competent colleague to carry out the manual task of actually undertaking the writing. Or, alternatively, the change agent is the motivator required to make the change happen, the driving force towards completion of the task. The person must be carefully selected in order to meet the needs of the role.

Finally, how to bring about the change? Having assembled all the other ingredients you now require a definite plan of action based upon sound knowledge of present practice. Write down the present system, as shown in the example in Figure 3.1. List all the various finite parts

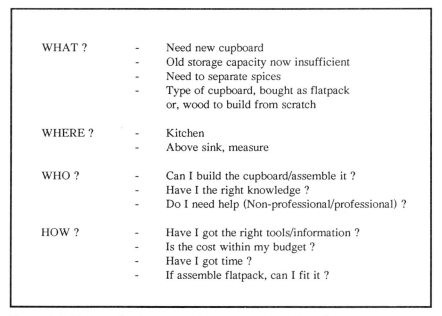

WHAT ?	-	Need new cupboard
	-	Old storage capacity now insufficient
	-	Need to separate spices
	-	Type of cupboard, bought as flatpack or, wood to build from scratch
WHERE ?	-	Kitchen
	-	Above sink, measure
WHO ?	-	Can I build the cupboard/assemble it ?
	-	Have I the right knowledge ?
	-	Do I need help (Non-professional/professional) ?
HOW ?	-	Have I got the right tools/information ?
	-	Is the cost within my budget ?
	-	Have I got time ?
	-	If assemble flatpack, can I fit it ?

Figure 3.1 Listing of points example, using cupboard analogy.

of a task and what other factors are involved. Consult with interested parties as to whether this is an accurate record of the present system.

When you have completed all the above, you should be ready to move on to the next stage.

Design requirements of the new system

From examining the present system, there should be something upon which you can base the future system. The earlier concept is also taken into account at this stage. Part of the design process is to plan a schedule of events, such as that shown in Figure 3.2. The schedule should be realistic and allow for consultation and adaptation. It will also show the short- and medium-term goals to be achieved, and it is always advantageous to have 'congratulatory' points during the change as a morale booster. The design stages will identify where change to present equipment or personnel is required.

If all the previous stages have been appropriately completed, it is often the case that this design part is the easiest, for decisions will have been made, albeit subconsciously, during the build-up to this point.

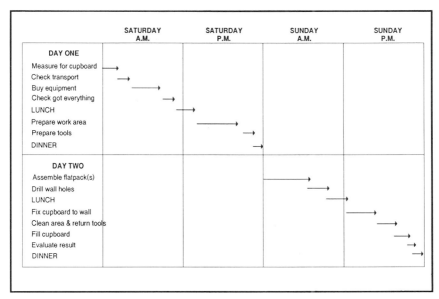

Figure 3.2 Schedule of events, cupboard assembly.

Implementation of the new system

This is possibly the simplest of all. You know why you want it, you know what you want, you know where you want it, you know who is going to do it and you know how it is going to be done! Unfortunately, you cannot just sit back and 'let it happen', for you must carefully watch each stage of development and be on hand to alter the system if an insurmountable problem occurs. Alteration or deviation from the plan includes considering the implications of such a move. For example, if during the screen design stage what you view is not quite what you had imagined, you can have discussions with everyone involved to try to ensure that your planned idea is still feasible, and that any changes to your plan are made without detriment to the educational value of the package.

Evaluation

This really begins during the previous stage, but when the new system has been implemented an overall evaluation is required. The timescale for commencement of an 'end' evaluation largely depends upon the task in hand; it may be immediate, or within a week, a month or a year. During the analysis stage, the criteria for the present system will have been assembled, and these should now be considered against the new system to note if it is successful.

Any change to a computer system, be it a wordprocessor (Chapter 4), or a larger nursing system for use either in the clinical or community area (Chapter 5), is exactly the same. The difficulty has often been that we have not been involved in early decision-making processes and thus have little or no feelings of ownership towards the new system. Perhaps if we understood more in the area of computing, then we might be able to assert ourselves and add our own already formed knowledge base (nursing) to the greater whole. What we have to offer as nurses, cannot be found anywhere else within the Health Service and as more and more ward-based systems are being implemented we should be there and involved in every stage.

Chapter Four

Computer applications in general

This chapter will cover the development and uses of 'content-free' computer applications for everyday use, such as databases, wordprocessing, spreadsheets and authoring tools. In order to understand the difference between using, for example, a wordprocessor and an electronic typewriter, we must consider the difference between mechanizing and computerizing.

For the purposes of this book, mechanization is considered to be the transfer of a task from a manual base to that of an electronic base, and, computerization is considered to be the transference from a manual set of tasks to the use of electronic tools for information interchange. The difficulty is that all too often computers are used within a mechanized framework rather than in fully developed computerization.

It is common for clerical staff, competent in the use of electronic typewriters, to be suddenly given computers with printers to replace their previous machines. Housed within the computer is a wordprocessor and the expectation of managers appears to be that the clerical staff will easily transfer from one form of typed output to another. However, very rarely is the transfer smooth, competent or well received by the clerical staff. Certainly a wordprocessor can be used like a typewriter and the keyboard is similar to that of a typewriter, but the power of the wordprocessor far exceeds that of a typewriter, as many competent users will agree. So why the belief that through the installation of computers computerization occurs?

Possibly one reason for such a belief is the use of the word 'computer', which conjures up a picture of processing power, of logical working practices and of a technical environment, yet computer implementation seldom ensures an analysis of working practices, which is the key to computerization. It should not be considered, however, that working practices should change to meet the needs of computer implementation, but the opportunity to examine traditional ways of working with traditional tools and systems should not be missed. The exercise of purchasing computers and the associated peripherals is costly but relatively easy in a market flush with the hardware to meet every need and keen salespeople around every corner. The exercise of unpacking the boxes and placing the computers on desks is often undertaken by the salespeople, so again it is easy for the purchaser. The exercise of ensuring that these costly tools are used to their full potential is another matter and seemingly one that is expected to occur through forcing individuals to use the computers, often without adequate training.

The same can be seen wherever computers are used in the Health Service. What has actually happened is that a previous manual system of work has been transferred to computer and the users mechanically go through their knowledge base in order to get out of the computer the information required, frequently not as they would wish to receive it, but to the best of their ability.

One only has to attend a 'computer training session' to see where the crux of the problem lies. The problem has come about due to lack of knowledge of information requirements over and above that of working practices prior to computer and system purchase. The training session generally contains a set of tasks that the user is taught, including which keys to press to obtain the required response from the computer, but quite whose 'required response' is often unclear. Surely this is mechanical training? Surely this will not advance computerization in the workplace? Surely this could be considered deskilling of previously highly competent personnel, both professional and support staff? Surely this is not an effective way forward for an organization? It is of course possible that even with massive computer investment in, for example, the Health Service, the requirement is for mechanized use. To be totally cynical, this would ensure that the required information output was gained but with no cognitive development of staff, ensuring that few pertinent questions were raised. How often does the excuse 'Sorry, the computer must have been faulty, that's why your salary slip doesn't include . . .' still meet with acceptance? How often does the point 'Oh no, the computer can't do . . .' meet with acceptance?

Too often we, the mere users of these powerful devices, meet with defensive answers from others nearer and more in tune with the technical powers of computers. The reason we frequently back away thinking 'There must be a way of doing . . . , but obviously that wasn't it' could be due to our own set traditional methods of working, our lack of knowledge of information flow through computer application tools such as wordprocessing, databases and spreadsheets, and an inherent fear of 'rocking the boat'. The latter is outside the remit of this book, but it is hoped that the reader is already some way down the road towards understanding the true meaning of computerization at this juncture and that the remaining chapters will further advance understanding.

Taking into account the above discussion, we should now examine why there is growing interest in the use of computers within the Health

Service. It is considered that by 1991 the Health Service had spent around £2 billion in computer developments and is currently spending around £50 million a year buying in computer and information tech nology consultancy to develop and rectify computer systems. What has been the driving force behind the development of computers and infor mation technology resulting in the sort of investment already made?

Much of the present interest in the use of technology for information storage, retrieval and dissemination stems from the publication of the Körner Reports (1984). Before the reports' development, health authorities would make returns covering all aspects of in- and out-patient statistics and other relevant figures to the Department of Health in a nonuniform manner. As can be imagined, the wealth of information was often lost, leaving decision-making in a somewhat dubious stance.

The Körner Reports suggested that more effective systems could be introduced and the recommendations from the reports have been taken up by health authorities across the country. They accept that there are differing levels of information needs in the NHS; for example, decision-making at national level may not require the same information needed at district level. To quote from the report's general approach:

'. . . we propose that routine collection of a series of minimum data sets to provide, at reasonable cost, the basic information without which authorities and their officers will not be adequately informed when fulfilling their responsibilities; we concentrate on identifying the information needs of the district health authority and its officers on the assumption that information not required for operational and for the district's own purposes will not normally be required regionally or nationally; the reliability and timeliness of data improve if they are collected as a by-product of operational procedures.'

NHS/DHSS Steering Group on Health Service Information,
Chairman: Mrs E. Körner, 1984

In taking the approach that districts should be the base level for information requirements the Körner recommendations certainly assist in a devolved service, with the knowledge base at district level. However, they do also recognize, as John Donne put it that 'no man is an island' and with information flow to and from district level in a meaningful form, greater understanding and co-ordination of developments can ensue from a regional or national level. The reports do not state that the information needs to be stored using computers, but it would appear that many health authorities looked to computerization and have developed computer systems to meet the demands of the Körner Report. Such systems have tended to reflect traditional working practices, even down to screen design mirroring the previous forms which were used to collect the same data manually. The reasons for the use of computers to perform the previous manual tasks are many, but one key factor is that through having information on a computer it can generally be quickly and easily retrieved which is vital for the busy manager today.

The *Working for Patients* (1988) series of government white papers has resulted in an information need by health service managers, and this too has furthered the development of computers and information technology in the Health Service. Much of the information required stems from the patient-contact areas (wards, departments or community) and nurses are involved as information providers and users. The next chapter considers the implications of the white paper *Working Paper 10* and of the nurses' role in the light of government changes and of systems already in operation.

In 1987, the Data Protection Act (1984) became fully operational, and it has major implications for the access by individuals to information stored about them. Health service systems take this into account during the design stage, for material sent out from the computer must be in a form that is understood by the individual, and must not divulge anything pertaining to any other individual. Even today discussion about the act is still going on, for it is expected that until a number of legal test cases have been heard the full implications will remain unknown.

CONTENT-FREE COMPUTING

A major breakthrough in the use of computers came with the development of content-free applications and packages. Some of these are more commonly referred to in their generic form as databases, wordprocessors and spreadsheets. Other more sophisticated systems and packages known as 'content-free shells' are available, but here we shall concentrate on the three first mentioned with one addition, that of authoring tools for use in education. As stated earlier, movement in the computer industry has progressively been towards freedom for the end user — freedom from coming to terms with 'actual computing', being able to use their own knowledge in whatever subject area, and finding an application tool to suit their needs.

The key to content-free computing is the development of information by the user. And the key to the development of information is required output; that is, users must have some idea of their information output requirements prior to selecting and using the appropriate application tool. The first common 'information processing' tool using a computer is generally wordprocessing, which permits the manipulation of textual information into a form required by the user, usually with limited predetermination of the eventual output, but with manipulation of the text following input into the final form. Other application tools, such as databases and spreadsheets, require predetermination of output prior to use and are thus more complex 'information processors', where prethought and design of information output is paramount. The same is true of authoring tools in education and training. There is little point in using any of the application tools unless information output meets identified need. It is not a case of using a tool merely for the sake of using a computer, for such ill-considered use tends to lead to frustration and disenchantment with the powerful computer device. The concept is the same for any of those tools mentioned above.

Consideration will now be given to databases and spreadsheets in a little detail. We shall then look briefly at wordprocessing and finally at authoring tools.

Database Application/Package

A database is a collection of information within a framework determined either by the user when using a PC, or by others when considering larger, more complex, collections of information. A database 'file' is made up of 'records' and each record contains 'fields' of information as shown in Figure 4.1. Prior to using a database four fundamental questions must be addressed.

1. Why are you setting up a database?
2. What information do you want in the database?
3. Who will use and have access to the database?

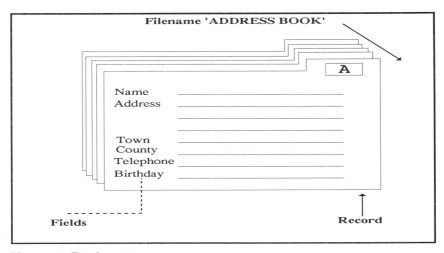

Figure 4.1 Database items.

4. What is the purpose of the database?

Having answered these questions and armed yourself with a computer and relevant peripherals, let us suppose that you have identified a need to store, analyse and retrieve data; for example an address list of friends. You now require a database package. The selection of a database application package is an easier solution that writing a program for a database and in most cases serves the purpose effectively.

The data to be stored could be:

1. surname
2. first name(s)
3. title (e.g. Mr, Mrs, Lord)
4. address
5. telephone number
6. birthday
7. card sent at Christmas.

Assessment must be made of the potential number of entries, for you do not want to run out of room before completing the list. How many address lines do you require and would you like a separate one for the postcode? Yes, we are back to analysis. Let's assume you have the information. After looking at a selection of databases, or after discussion with others, you find a suitable application package.

The package must permit you to enter the information in a form suitable for you, to change, delete or add information at a later date; to analyse the information depending upon your chosen criteria; and to obtain paper copies in a form meaningful and useful to you.

Having mastered the art of turning on the computer and loading the appropriate package you are now ready to input the information. Most database systems work on a series of menus, which are generally explained in an accompanying manual. From experience, it is well worth having a practice run following an initial reading of the documentation. Then off you go. When all the information is in, it may be the case that the surnames are not in alphabetical order, but sorting is generally possible from a menu selection.

Large computer systems with databases work along very similar lines, the main difference being in the design of the format, as this may have been decided prior to implementation and thus your use.

Owing to a need to develop information systems that link information in some form, in recent times the phrase 'data modelling' has appeared in our vocabulary. The key element of this, over and above our examination of systems thinking, is the relationships of pieces of data to each other and to outside factors. Data modelling, as the name suggests, is the art of building a suitable model to handle and manipulate information in a way that meets the given goal. It may include collections of specific data elements to satisfy another data area; for example the number of people attending hospital for surgery needs to be added to all other admission types to give the total admissions but it may be necessary to know the surgical figures alone for future theatre scheduling.

Each area of data is called a 'file', a number of files may relate to one item of information, and within each file are 'records', such as one set of details pertaining to one individual. Within each individual's record are 'fields'; for example title of the person, (Mr, Mrs, Miss, or Ms). These files have a common purpose, that of fulfilling an information need, and a field relationship here would be that of relating gender to title.

We can liken the principle of information fields to that of left luggage lockers commonly found at railway and bus stations and airports. Each locker represents a file, the size is variable to incorporate the differing sizes of luggage, and yet all are designed for one specific purpose. Users choose the locker most suitable for their needs, follow the outlined procedure and secure their possessions for retrieval at a later time.

A difference between static lockers and data modelling is the determination of relationships between the files. Continuing with the luggage metaphor, when travelling by airplane a passenger's luggage is identified by attached labels, and although only one collection point may be in existence, the label recognition permits sorting of the luggage on to the corresponding flight, thus luggage is luggage, but the relationship is luggage-to-passenger-to-flight. An example in nursing terms of data modelling is given in the next chapter. The content is an important factor in developing any system. The requirements must be determined before design stages are reached; working through relationship data modelling is an excellent method of determining the content need required by a variety of end users, both those putting the information in and those who will take the information out. Figure 4.2 identifies the in – out relationships involved in the design of a system for information concerning continuing education for nursing staff. The basic information is used by a wide range of people within the organization, so an obvious pay-off from such a single information store is the reduction in duplication, indeed in many instances, triplication.

The concept of data modelling is that of reduction in effort whilst improving the quality (and possibly quantity) of data for information. With computer developments, we have the facility of 'shells' into which the required content for the data fits. The shell also permits access to the data in order to use the information as a tool for improved management of our respective working environments.

With databases, it is imperative that any personal data is protected and, if appropriate, the database is registered under the requirements

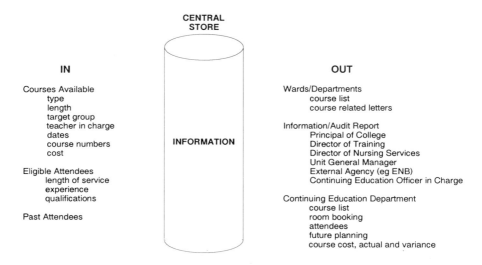

CENTRAL
STORE

IN

Courses Available
  type
  length
  target group
  teacher in charge
  dates
  course numbers
  cost

Eligible Attendees
  length of service
  experience
  qualifications

Past Attendees

INFORMATION

OUT

Wards/Departments
  course list
  course related letters

Information/Audit Report
  Principal of College
  Director of Training
  Director of Nursing Services
  Unit General Manager
  External Agency (eg ENB)
  Continuing Education Officer in Charge

Continuing Education Department
  course list
  room booking
  attendees
  future planning
  course cost, actual and variance

Figure 4.2 Input and output using a central store of core information.

of the Data Protection Act. The main points of the act are listed at the
back of the book.

Spreadsheet Application/Package

As with the database package, users add their own content to an application tool/shell already designed. A spreadsheet is a large matrix with
two main axes, each one generally consisting of 255 columns and rows,
and therefore containing over 65,000 individual boxes or cells. Because
of its enormous size the whole sheet cannot be displayed on one screen,
so the user is generally presented with 'window' presenting part of the
sheet. Movement to other sections of the spreadsheet is easily achiev-
able. Spreadsheets have a basis firmly in mathematics. For those without leanings in this direction, this could be the tool for you to use!

In order to explain the system, an example of a potential educational
requirement will be used, that is the marks assigned to work following
the assessment of twelve learners for a period of one year. We shall
assume that during the year, each student must write three essays and
present a piece of individual project work, all of which go towards their
end-of-year assessment which must reach a minimum pass of 55%.
In addition, the student is offered the opportunity of assessing their
knowledge retrieval through a marked multiple choice paper, but this
figure is not part of the year-end total.

The first stage is to set up the framework of the spreadsheet for the
function required as shown in Figure 4.3. The relationship of the boxes

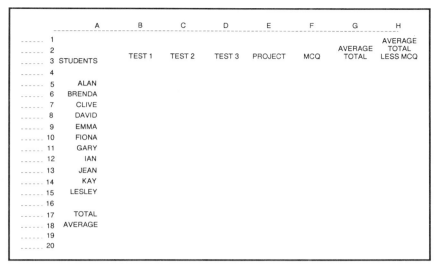

Figure 4.3 Spreadsheet template.

is devised (data modelling), that is, all the entries in column B will be added together to form a total at the bottom. B4 to B15 added together and divided by 12 gives the average total marks for that essay for the group. Similarly, the rows across need to be added together B4 + C4 + D4 + E4 divided by 4 (shown in H4) gives the average total for each individual. We can add the multiple choice result to a different average total if we wish; B4 + C4 + D4 + E4 + F4 divided by 5 (shown in G4).

Once satisfied with the relationships of the columns and rows, the actual marks can be inserted as shown in Figure 4.4. In a conscious effort to repeat the information processing premise, the setting up and predetermination of information output is all-important; once it has been done the actual implementation on to the computer is simple.

On the spreadsheet is now a massive amount of data that can be interpreted as required. Not only does it show the individual performance of students, it shows at a glance the overall validity of the questions asked in the bottom total. If there were clearly visible fluctuations along this bottom line, concern might be raised as to the validity of the question posed, or indeed the marker's assessment of the students' answers.

As with any 'content-free' package, the uses and complexity of design of such an application tool grow as users develop their own knowledge of the application tool. The example shown is only the tip of the spreadsheet iceberg, but perhaps encourages thought in the potential uses of such an application tool.

	A	B	C	D	E	F	G	H
1								AVERAGE
2							AVERAGE	TOTAL
3	STUDENTS	TEST 1	TEST 2	TEST 3	PROJECT	MCQ	TOTAL	LESS MCQ
4								
5	ALAN	46.Ø	72.Ø	64.Ø	79.Ø	56.Ø	63.4	65.3
6	BRENDA	78.Ø	65.Ø	59.Ø	67.Ø	73.Ø	68.4	67.3
7	CLIVE	67.Ø	80.Ø	86.Ø	72.Ø	57.Ø	72.4	76.3
8	DAVID	56.Ø	62.Ø	65.Ø	64.Ø	78.Ø	65.Ø	61.8
9	EMMA	89.Ø	78.Ø	69.Ø	75.Ø	64.Ø	75.Ø	77.8
10	FIONA	64.Ø	60.Ø	62.Ø	62.Ø	63.Ø	62.2	62.Ø
11	GARY	67.Ø	59.Ø	52.Ø	53.Ø	55.Ø	57.2	57.8
12	IAN	70.Ø	74.Ø	78.Ø	72.Ø	68.Ø	72.4	73.5
13	JEAN	34.Ø	54.Ø	54.Ø	40.Ø	32.Ø	42.8	45.5
14	KAY	78.Ø	61.Ø	65.Ø	66.Ø	71.Ø	68.2	67.5
15	LESLEY	69.Ø	64.Ø	66.Ø	70.Ø	69.Ø	67.6	67.3
16								
17	TOTAL							
18	AVERAGE	65.3	66.3	65.5	65.5	62.4		
19								
20								

Figure 4.4 Spreadsheet with contents added.

Wordprocessing Application/Package

The wordprocessor is a system based upon the requirements of those generally working in secretarial support services and for personal use at home. Most wordprocessing systems are based upon the 'QWERTY' keyboard known and loved by all. Voice-activated wordprocessors are being developed, but although some demonstration models are already around it is likely to be some time before these become generally available; thus the more traditional method of keyboard input will be considered.

There is no one national standard wordprocessor, each manufacturer having brought out their own, or versions of a common core wordprocessor. However the principles of use are generally the same. Some computers are 'dedicated' wordprocessors; that is all they do. Other wordprocessors are additions to the computer which means that the computer can be used for computing functions as well as wordprocessing although generally not at the same time! Mainframe and minicomputers are capable of a number of different functions at any one time, but in most cases wordprocessing is performed on microcomputers.

Many users state that a wordprocessor is an intelligent typewriter, in that the user can choose format, position of text, make alterations and print out material (hard copy) in a way meaningful to them. There is often a rigorous training period needed to understand fully the strengths and pitfalls of the wordprocessor being used. In talking to people who frequently use these systems it seems that they believe that all staff should understand the basic principles involved, so that the most efficient method of use can be obtained.

Advantages of wordprocessors are many, but include the ability to proof-read material prior to producing hard copy. Editing becomes a less tedious task in that often only parts of the document require changing and not all of it needs to be retyped. There is always a perfect end hard copy (no white 'blobs' highlighting earlier errors) and with standard letters a merging system can be used to link a database of addresses to the text, so that each letter is personalized. In addition, frequently supplied with the wordprocessor package is a spelling check dictionary and sometimes a thesaurus, although spelling is generally not 'content proof', in that 'their' would be correct whereas you may have meant 'there'. Entering the market now are grammar checkers linked to wordprocessors, but at the moment these tend to be expensive and have not been tested by the author.

Disadvantages of a wordprocessor include the user facing a screen all day and the possible health implications involved, although reports have been issued by certain trade unions denying the harmful effects advanced initially. There may be initial paper wastage as the system is learnt and on some systems the end result including different fonts (eg italics, underlining, etc.) cannot be viewed on the screen before printing out. Others, however, do show you an exact picture on screen of the eventual hard copy. These are known as WYSIWYG systems (What You See Is What You Get) and corrections may be made more frequently due to the ease of use.

As with any application tool, a wordprocessor is only as effective as the user's ability to use all aspects of the package. In everyday use many aspects of wordprocessing may not be frequently used. The method of use may be temporarily forgotten, leading to a reversion to complete retyping rather than identifying a more correct procedure. Learning about wordprocessing takes time and effort, even for an individual competent at using a typewriter, and the time commitment for learning will probably be around 20 hours split into taught and practice sessions. All will not be evident during a short initial course and continued learning is required which often includes reinforcement of aspects not commonly used. Here is a plea to those instigating work for input on to a wordprocessor. This is a complex tool and requires a sound knowledge base by the user; if this is understood a good working relationship should ensue.

Additions for wordprocessor packages may include some form of data storage system, for names and addresses for example, that can be merged with the main package to save time and effort. As mentioned above, a spelling check package is usually available and although this often takes time to set up for individually required words it does ensure that most documents will leave the system with no spelling errors. Some systems permit the use of different fonts, that is, the type of printed characters used. For example it is possible to change from a commonly used print face to italic print face without changing pieces of paper. The wordprocessor has revolutionized the office environment, but it is worth remembering that this application tool, as with any computer tool, is only as good as its user.

Authoring application tools/packages

The final area of 'content-free' computing which should be discussed focuses on the educational use of the computer, that is, authoring application tools.

There are a variety of authoring tools available; in varying formats, ROM or disc-based, and at various prices. The point of an authoring tool is that the framework is already built for you; all the user does in terms of computing or programming is to input the content required.

In developing a learning program for students, the wish of educationists would be to motivate and increase the knowledge of students in a given area of the curriculum, thus adding to their overall developing professional knowledge base through another medium. The subject material, the flow of that material and its place in the curriculum must be thoroughly considered and developed before transferring it to the computer authoring tool, possibly through using a chart similar to that shown in Figure 4.5, which considers all the variables involved in the subject area. Other factors which will require consideration will include where text, graphics or questions will be used, and possible multiple answers to each question.

Having achieved a satisfactory draft of flow and content, the user loads the authoring tool and the creation of the package begins. Commonly the first screen will be that of the title page, followed by a menu choice of

1. text
2. graphics
3. question
4. end.

Users choose the next 'page' in relation to their flow chart. This may be text, followed by a graphical representation of the material (or section of the material), perhaps more text, then a question. Each of the selected

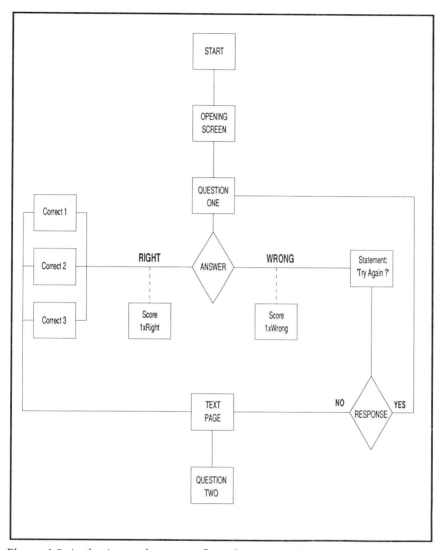

Figure 4.5 Authoring tool, content flow chart example.

'pages' is offered to the user by the computer and the content added in the way the user wishes.

With the question section, most authoring tools now facilitate a variety of answer formats including 'sounds like' (for those of us with spelling problems). The content author determines the number of tries at each question, the number of right or wrong answers, the statements to follow these if selected by the student, and so on. As has been mentioned, there is no computing in the classical sense at all; what is developed is the use of the technology and a useful tool, and as such it is educational for the content author as well as producing an end result for the curriculum.

Users take a while to become conversant with and fully appreciate authoring tools. As with the previous content-free application tools mentioned, their strength lies in the fact that to use a computer you do not need to understand a complicated programming language, but the creativity of use does depend upon the content-author's ability to use the tool effectively for educational purposes.

With many of the currently available authoring application tools, there is an editing section, which tends to resemble the more common programming languages (e.g. Figure 4.6). For those with greater techni-

---

This listing is taken from a short question section within a geography lesson, using the TopClass Authoring Tool (Format PC). The items in brackets are not part of the design, they are given as explanation to the abbreviated terms.

```
.SCR 1                              (Clear screen)
.PAL 1                              (Select background colour)
.COL 4                              (select text colour)
.LOCATE 10,0                        (text screen position)
        WORLD GEOGRAPHY
.LOCATE 12,0                        (text screen position for next line)
        LESSON ONE
.LOC 24,1                           (put in user instruction 'Space Bar')
.PAU                                (pause until space bar is pressed)
@BEGIN QUESTION 1
.CLS                                (clear screen)
@TRI 1                              (display first question)
        WHAT IS THE CAPITAL OF THE USA ?
@REA(*Your answer :*)              (awaiting a response)
@RIG(*WASHINGTON D.C.*) EXACT NOCASE
                                    (first right answer identified by teacher, the
                                    response can be either upper or lower case)
WELL DONE                           (teacher selected response to above)
@RIG(*WASHINGTON D C*) EXACT NOCASE
                                    (second identified right answer)
CORRECT, BUT SHOULD HAVE FULL STOPS AFTER THE D AND C
                                    (teacher selected response to right answer 2)
```

The actual program is considerably longer than shown above, however, the example does show the use of a high level language and relatively easy commands for program design.

Figure 4.6 Extract from question section.

cal bents, it is possible to use the editor to build the package rather than the content-free system. The editing section is also used to make minor amendments, most individuals seeming to enjoy the challenge of using this section once initial fear and apprehension is overcome.

It should be stressed that when designing any form of content-free application software for use, a team approach should be taken. The variety of knowledge and skills available should be fully used during the design and writing stages of the package, and this is particularly important for databases, spreadsheets and authoring tools.

Through examining briefly some of the major 'content-free' areas and developments it is hoped that readers will feel more at ease with their possible use of computers. In this day and age it is no longer necessary to understand the actual language of the computer. It is our responsibility to understand the uses we wish to make of this powerful tool, and this may involve using systems described here to get a 'feel' for the computer and its components. The content (use) of the computer is the vital area, not the make of computer, the number of terminals or standard systems. The content is the responsibility of the user and this must be taken into account whenever a computer system is under consideration. In the area of nursing, we are the content experts and this should never be forgotten.

In the next chapter some current uses of computers in nursing in the United Kingdom are considered, perhaps to serve to whet the reader's appetite!

Chapter Five

Computer applications in nursing: clinical, administrative and educational

Nursing involvement with computers in the United Kingdom dates back over two decades. In 1969, three projects were commenced to examine the possible role of computers in health care, although even these three had their roots in an earlier experiment at King's College Hospital, London. The projects were centrally funded and dispersed across the UK, and the sites chosen at Dundee, Birmingham and Exeter all had major responsibilities for forging links between health (clinical/community) environments and the technical computing environment. These early centres were quickly followed by others in the country, and through their work nurses were able to perceive the potential of ward-based computer systems.

Each centre developed a ward-based nursing system. The system concentrated upon the care plan section of clinical nursing and through the nurses' use, ward and patient workload/dependency estimations were obtained. Each ward typically had a visual display unit with a keyboard attached through cables to the main computer, usually a large mainframe. In some instances the ward also had a printer for obtaining hard copy documentation when required. The main computer was not solely for the use of the nursing system, and indeed many variable uses were often running concurrently, such as laboratory systems, general practitioner systems, in- and outpatient systems (medical records), finance and personnel.

In those early years, nursing was beginning to move away from task allocation to that of patient allocation, and the use of the computer went some way towards assisting this evolution in those centres cited above through the individuality of care plans. Nursing input was used from the beginning, and as the systems grew the importance of the clinical and educational nursing staff became generally recognized. Links were made between nurses and systems analysts in order that misconceptions could be reduced, language barriers broken and common ground established. Much of this work by those in at the beginning has helped ensure the position today. It is perhaps our conceptual abilities that held us back rather than an unwillingness to pursue the innovative path.

The main objectives for these projects were, according to Redmond (1983):

1. to ensure better patient care;
2. to increase clinical and administrative efficiency;
3. to improve management and research facilities.

As is clearly obvious, these were high aims for any innovation, but they did provide a core element or goal for achievement.

The 1970s sped by and many alterations to the systems were implemented and policy shifts adhered to by the centres. In 1977, a report, *A Review of Computing* (NHS/DHSS, 1977), was published proposing a devolution of the central control then exercised upon NHS computing. According to Redmond (1983),

'This in turn led to a complete re-evaluation of the way in which computing policy had been administered; and further, of how successful it had been.'

Indeed, there have been further changes and reports, the most important ones being from the Körner Committee (1984) and, more recently, from the NHS Management Board Information Advisory Group, *A National Strategic Framework for Information Management in the Hospital and Community Health Services* (1986), which was a precurser to the Government's white paper *Working for Patients* (1988). In the foreword to the NHS Management Board IAG's document the following comment is worthy of quotation.

'. . . the requirements for information are growing at every point in the service (NHS) and that technological advances now offer a myriad of ways to satisfy that demand . . . there is awareness of this opportunity and it is clear that expenditure in this area is growing rapidly. The danger is that the rising tide of IT (Information Technology), the pace of development and the excitement that flows with it, may surge uncontrollably through the Health Service. The framework seeks to ensure that we harness to maximum benefit the money and resource which the Health Service will be expending in this area in coming years.'

Fairey, 1986

Time having passed, perhaps it can be seen that the early sorties into the technological world for nursing systems were advanced beyond their times; the results from the three earlier cited centres demonstrated that computers could be used as an integral part of a ward management system. '. . . *they also helped to create a wide range of expertise in health care computing, thus providing a base for the future.*' (Redmond, 1983)

It was no longer a question of should we use computers, but how are we going to use them. We have perhaps gone further than we think down the path of achieving the goals set out in the late 1960s and early 1970s, as Ball and Hannah (1984) state;

> 'The strength of nursing depends upon its ability to take advantage of the best that modern technology can offer. This implies that information will be used to further enhance clinical nursing practice, to support administrative decision making, to facilitate nursing education and expand the body of nursing knowledge through research.'

The following examination of some of the present uses of computers in nursing is considered as an overview. It is inappropriate in this book to present a more complete picture, or do justice to the hard work and effort involved in producing such systems, for which apologies are given. A resource list is included in the references where further explanation of the uses can be found.

The systems in use in the UK can be broadly defined into three categories: clinical, administrative and educational. It must be stated that the boundaries between these categories are often clouded, although the educational element is certainly evident in all the uses, for through developing and handling any computer system learning takes place and thus progress ensues. The following systems identified will show approaches taken, references being given where appropriate.

CLINICAL

As we stated earlier, ward-based clinical nursing systems are in evidence in the UK at a number of centres; they have grown in complexity with advancing knowledge of computers and with the use of data modelling. One such model is shown in Figure 5.1. The use of systematic thinking is evident in order to obtain the model and the relationships between various identified factors are taken into consideration.

As can be seen, the model is highly sophisticated and contains a vast amount of historical data. The relevant points have been determined by experienced nurses with a nurse leader steering the discussions.

> 'The relevant problems for the patient are selected, the system can then highlight "problem complications" related to the interaction of two separately identified problems. In other words the rules are stored in the "complicating factor" function area. A simple example is if the problem box for continence indicates that a patient is incontinent and the problem box for mobility indicates that the patient is

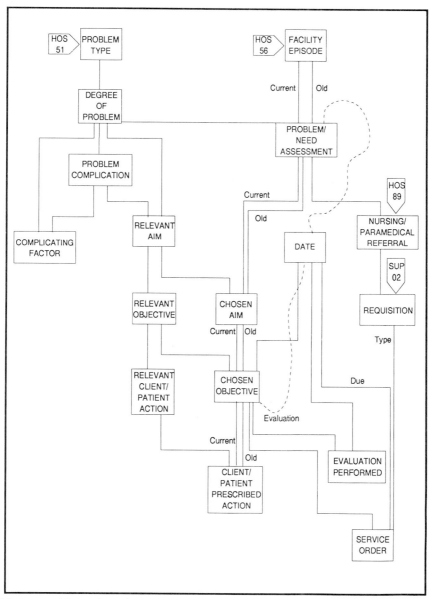

Figure 5.1 Flow chart for nursing system (Adapted from Roberts and Taylor, 1987).

immobile, these create a potential problem for the patient who might develop pressure sores. Appropriate preventative action must then be taken. Using the data models has identified that modifications may be necessary and that some of the definitions require clarification or expansion . . .'

Roberts and Taylor 1987

Many levels of staff have been involved in developing this model and certainly the planners believe that a continual evaluative approach needs to be undertaken, thus allowing for flexibility in a complex situation. A problem in the past has been the belief that a computer system cannot accurately reflect the changing needs of patient care in the naturally dynamic clinical situation, but to some degree these problems have been overcome with a flexible system such as the one shown.

In most ward-based systems currently being used, the additional management information is not gleaned through the normal everyday use of the system with additional work on the part of the nurse, and thus these systems tend not to be valued operationally. A variety of finance and workload/dependency estimators are in evidence, some more accurate than others. However, the major output of all of them is that quantifiable data is obtained quickly. Figure 5.2 is an example of dependency estimations collected for one ward for one month, based on the Barr 5 (1972) categorization.

Some of the ward-based systems are directly linked to the Patient Administration System (PAS), which is a logical connection. The admitting nurse is able to check if the patient has previously been to the hospital, thus reducing duplication of notes and inaccuracies in hospital patient statistics. It must be stated that this is not true in a large number of currently used systems, and perhaps it should be. Where such an interlink has occurred it has proved particularly useful where the PAS information is retrievable in an accident and emergency department.

Other clinical systems include 'loop-feedback' programs, which have found a secure home especially in intensive care/therapy units. An example of one such system is in the use of a specific anti-inflammatory drug in cases where there is cerebral oedema. The system operates rather like the nervous system's reflex arc. The computer is the central element and an electrode is suitably placed in the patient's bloodstream measuring changes in the pressure exerted through the oedema quickly and accurately. This electrode sends information to the computer, the medical staff having previously determined the parameters of dose-to-pressure reading and stored the variables in the computer. When information is received by the computer from the electrode, the computer checks its program and initiates the appropriate amount of the drug to be administered, in a continual process. The results have been

The following patient dependency estimations are based upon the Barr 5 (1972) categorisation.

DAY	Patients	Group 1	Group 2	Group 3	Group 4	Group 5	Average Total
1	26	5	Ø	9	7	5	3.27
2	24	3	1	11	6	3	3.21
3	27	4	1	8	1Ø	4	3.33
4	2Ø	2	1	5	7	5	3.6Ø
5	21	3	1	5	8	4	3.43
6	26	3	1	5	9	4	3.38
7	27	3	1	1Ø	9	4	3.37
8	27	3	2	14	5	3	3.11
9	27	4	2	13	5	3	3.Ø4
10	26	3	3	9	9	2	3.15
11	22	2	3	9	7	2	3.14
12	23	4	3	7	7	2	3.ØØ
13	24	4	3	9	6	2	2.96
14	25	4	2	1Ø	6	3	3.Ø8
15	22	4	2	5	7	4	3.23
16	25	6	2	3	9	5	3.2Ø
17	27	7	2	4	9	5	3.11
18	24	5	2	4	8	5	3.25
19	22	3	2	4	8	5	3.45
2Ø	25	3	2	1Ø	4	6	3.32

Brief Group Summary:

Group 1	A patient who requires minimal support
Group 2	A partial care patient who requires some help and supervision
Group 3	A medium care patient, requiring nursing staff to initiate, supervise or perform most activities
Group 4	A total care patient, conscious or unconscious
Group 5	A patient requiring intensive care/one nurse constantly

The Barr 5 categorisation was an early dependency framework, and as such it is not based on any current 'nursing model', but is given as a statistical example.

Figure 5.2 Example of patient dependency estimations (20 days).

most encouraging from such systems and the mortality rate has reduced dramatically in most cases where it has been used. The traditional method of 'bolus' doses certainly did not have the same effect. Other 'loop-feedback' systems include neonatal monitoring systems which observe changes in breathing patterns, and then give a stimulus to the newborn infant to induce the expected breathing pattern.

Another area of development has been that of ward-based drug-prescribing systems which, although in the medical staff domain, is certainly an asset to nurses. One such system uses a minicomputer with terminals (VDU, keyboard and printer) on the ward. Using the terminal the medical practitioner selects the patient for whom the new drug is required. The computer relays information already stored on the patient's present drug regime, the medical practitioner selects the drug required and the computer checks its data banks for contra-indications in relation to the regime already in operation, informs the medical practitioner of any of these, and in some cases suggests a cheaper alternative that does the same job.

If the doctor is unsure of the route, dosage or frequency of the drug the computer will relay that information upon request. When the prescribing medical practitioner is satisfied that the new regime is correct a revised hard copy printout is obtained. This printout is used by the nursing staff when administering the drug to the patient.

In any clinical system where patient information is contained in printed form a strict policy ensuring confidentiality is always maintained, usually through the issuing of passwords or 'log-in codes'. Each person with a right to access information from the computer is issued with a unique coded password. The password is checked by the computer and access to the relevant area permitted. It is the responsibility of the password holder to ensure that no one else uses their code. A password system as described above is rather like the use made of identity numbers for bank service till cards. It is unfortunate that at the time of writing it is understood that the Department of Health does not accept the use of unique computer password identity codes from a legal perspective; it is hoped that such a stance will be amended in the near future.

On the same theme of confidentiality, any documentation containing patient information is carefully stored, and once no longer required is destroyed following agreed policies. In the case of records that must be kept for a given time period, these are often stored following transfer of the paper copy to microfiche medium. The microfiche system used is similar to that found in some libraries, where a specialized viewer is used and the microfiche 'slide' is enlarged in order that the user can read the information. Microfiche storage permits large amounts of data to be retained in a small and unobtrusive space.

All systems used for patient data have full back-up facilities. This is required in case of system failure and generally the storage medium is tape. The back up should be stored in a different place from the main 'in-use' or 'live' data system, in case of fire damage. Generally systems automatically back themselves up at given time points during the day, which involves in some instances the live system being inoperable for that back-up period. It is vitally important that such a disaster-recovery policy is built into any computer developments that involve live system use.

NURSING ADMINISTRATION

There has been much advancement in the use of computers in this area, with all manner of tools implemented to assist the nurse managers at all levels to obtain the information they require to fulfil their role.

The workload/dependency estimations already briefly mentioned have resulted in more efficient determination of manpower requirements and ward/department establishments. As stated, these may not give all the information required, but they do go a long way towards setting standards within the nurse managers' domain which can be measured for attainment. A number of these systems, still in their infancy, use a paper method of data collection. The data is then fed into a computer and the resulting information is relayed to the manager and the ward or department. Trends can be easily seen, and with continued use more data will become available so that effective planning can be undertaken in relation to manpower requirements. Figure 5.3 is an example of graphical representation of the workload data shown in Figure 5.2.

Staffing is one of the major areas in nursing management, so it is fitting that this area is one of growth in the development of computer tools. The range of systems is expanding from basic personnel systems to staff scheduling systems; indeed, integrated systems relating ward/department workload-to-employed personnel-to-scheduling systems are beginning to emerge.

Personnel systems are databases with all the required information on staff employed. This method of storage is potentially safer than that of cards or files, in that unique password entry is generally employed, and the responsibility for security and confidentiality rests with the password holder. It is understood that it is a relatively simple task to break into a filing cabinet or office, but it can be considerably more

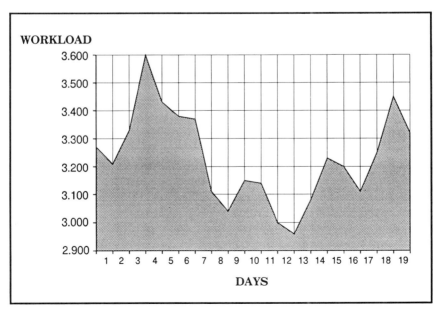

Figure 5.3 Graph of data in Figure 5.2.

difficult to break into a password-controlled computer system if it has been designed with thought.

A personal example of this springs to mind. Picture if you will a cold January Friday at 6.30p.m. I am not in my home town and, needing cash for an evening out, I place my card in the bank service till and insert what I think is my unique identity code, only to find it is the wrong number . . . Two attempts left before losing the card, panic sets in . . . previous use had been so simple . . . take card out, think, re-attempt, wrong number . . . think again, queue forming, try last attempt, wrong . . . card gone, no money, walk away dejected.

Information is the key to management and the manipulation of that information is the skill of management. Obtaining the information can frequently be time-consuming and tedious, but a number of systems using computers have arrived to relieve the information-handling pro-cess. The fundamental aspect of all management systems is that the information held on them must be meaningful and helpful to the man-ager.

A system in operation in some health districts in the community section does assist with the individual's reduction in time-consuming administrative duties. The community nurse maintains the clients' records using a hand-held computer database, with access available to that community nurse alone. In some of these systems, much of the input is coded to reduce input time, but the nurse can detail as much as required for each client; in others very few codes are used. The computer can also act as a diary for visits, a reference for addresses and reason for visit, with the data stored showing the GP's details and, if initiated, many other useful data areas. Upon completion of the visits, the nurse returns to the centre and, using a modem link, uploads the information for that day on to a main computer or alternatively to a single computer with a large memory store for linkage to a main central system later. Thus the information stored from a number of community nurses can be correlated and decision-making made easier for the com-munity nurse manager.

In health visiting, a system in development deals with prioritizing case loads. A number of parameter indices are set, based upon past researched work in the health visiting area and related to input details of the cases of each health visitor (HV). The system also permits the HV to input future dates when revisits are required, and these appear on the case load diary at the appropriate date and time. The trials of the system have shown that the planning and administrative work of the HV has been reduced and that the priority cases are always flagged for visits.

Not yet mentioned, but underlying all administration systems, is the management of often scarce resources. In these cost-conscious days, there is an increasing awareness of the adequate use of scarce resources both human and financial. Manpower planning systems frequently have a financial element already integrated into the system, and this is very useful for the nurse manager. In many instances though, the reality of the situation is that such resource management systems have not had nursing input in their design stage and thus are often meaningless to the nurse managers for whom they are meant. It is not very useful to be told if one is over- or under-spent without a clear indication of how the spending relates to the manager's budget. Instances are known where the actual target budget figure is not known by the nurse managers and this leads to a feeling of lack of control in their environment. It is imperative that nurses gain involvement at an early stage of system development in order the autonomy can be preserved and fully attained later when using a system.

With the systems mainly installed for resource management initiatives there is another difficulty for nursing generally, in that if an attempt to add a 'nursing' section is visible it is generally tagged on to the end of the main system and in many cases is both educationally and practically unsound.

In administration, computerization can either be a blessing or a hindrance. Those to whom it is a blessing are frequently those who have been actively involved in developing a system; those to whom it is a hindrance tend to be those for whom no involvement was forthcoming.

EDUCATION

The use of computers in education has grown dramatically since 1983, in both general secondary schools and colleges and in nursing education. Much of the future of nurses' use of computers and information technology will depend upon the way in which computers are introduced in nursing education. It is hoped that through recent national projects, such as the English National Board's Computer Assisted Learning Project (1988–91), computers and information technology are being integrated across curricula and are not viewed as relevant to specific curriculum areas or used solely for distinct package education or remedial activities. There are a variety of uses open to curriculum integration and educational administration, some of which are highlighted below.

The maintenance of student training records is now nearly all on computer, particularly where the statutory bodies are concerned. Use of computers as an educational tool has been recognized by teachers for some time, but creative use of the tool has been slow in developing in the UK. Through the efforts of enthusiasts and those committed to the computer tool in education, many packages are available covering a variety of curriculum aspects. They are generally concerned with one specific topic area, for example blood grouping or explanation of relevant legislation ('content-fixed'). Most of them do tend towards the drill and practice method of instruction, but even these have a potential place in our changing education climate, for with some students there is a need to work repeatedly through an exercise before understanding is forthcoming.

Some more sophisticated progams are becoming available which actually 'educate' in the true sense of the word, in that they move the student on from what is known to what is unknown and then learnt. Some advantages of using computers in education from the students' point of view include the following.

1. Students set their own pace.
2. Self-study principles are generated.
3. Identification of other useful resources can be offered during a package related to in-house availability.
4. The program can be repeated as often as required.
5. There is a challenge to develop knowledge and skill in a given area.

Advantages from the teachers' point of view include the following.

1. The path the student follows in using the program can be identified, allowing for personal counselling or intervention.
2. The teacher is aware of what students have gone through in their learning.
3. A standard can be set in a topic area.

The disadvantages are generally concerned with the level of sophistication of the program and the relevance to the establishment's curriculum. Computer-assisted learning (CAL) packages are generally 'slotted' into curricula, which has often reinforced the view that the packages are remedial rather than educative.

A program that generated much interest was from St George's District School of Nursing, London (1988). In essence the program is a database of information relating to case histories of a number of unidentified patients. The program is used by the student prior to a discussion session. From going through the database, the student makes certain assumptions about the patient, which vary depending upon previous knowledge, experience and information given by the database. The author of the package has noted that the discussion sessions have covered more topic areas and been livelier than corresponding control groups who did not examine the database prior to the discussion session. One point also discovered was that the control group generally felt that the discussion had gone well and were satisfied with the outcome, whereas the computer group felt dissatisfied with the discussion, and wished more time had been allocated to come to reasonable conclusions. The computer group felt they had got more out of the discussion.

In post-basic education, a package that gained national recognition came from the collaboration of the Nightingale School, West Lambeth Health Authority and the University of Surrey. The package was designed to form a framework for content, which at the present time, is that of intravenous drug administration. It is aimed at all nursing staff with responsibility for such drug administration. A computer-selected patient scenario is given and the nurse then has to determine unprompted, but with help if requested, what further information it is necessary to obtain prior to safe administration of an intravenous drug. Following this an objective test is issued with two attempts permitted. A printout summarizing the nurse's progress and score is obtained which can be discussed with the tutor. However the level of sophistication of this package is most evident in the non-student areas. Some of the non-student areas of interest to cite here are the ability for tutors, through an editing facility, to make the subject content applicable to local drug policies and practices; using the same facility, tutors can change the level and priority of information to be gathered and questions to be answered; finally, tutors can view and print out a record of the student's progress through the package and the scores they obtained. To utilize fully the power of such a package requires detailed subject analysis and curriculum integration skills. As with all innovations, a degree of empiricism is essential.

It is interesting to note that in nursing and midwifery education the move away from 'drill and practice' programs is becoming evident, and indeed there are numerous packages now available that move the user from the known to the unknown in a cognitive manner. The change in use is certainly due to greater understanding of the computer as a tool for education rather than its past uses as an electronic 'page turner'.

Greater use of content-free tools is also being introduced, and this has the potential for increasing creative use of the computer in education and ultimately clinical practice; for example, wordprocessing for student projects, databases for relevant references and spreadsheets for student planning experimentation. Through educational uses of computers another, perhaps covert, achievement is a grounding of knowledge about the computer itself, which will grow during future years as more educational uses are found and more students use such packages and content-free application tools. The computer can do more than act as a remedial tool; for example, packages are available which increase group discussion during decision-making in response to triggers from the computer, where the teacher's role is that of observer of group dynamics and as an exterior resource for the student.

The computer in education should not be viewed as a replacement for teachers, more as a tool to aid teachers in educating their students. An example in this area concerns the use of a computer program giving a group of students information for a patient assessment, then displaying a preset list of nursing actions from which a selection is made. The chosen action causes changes to occur in the patient information, though these may not always be an immediate change to the patients' status. The students continue to give their chosen actions until they reach a satisfactory level shown in the patient information details. It is then determined whether the care chosen was suitable for the specified patient or not. In use with groups, this program has tended to cause much student discussion and on occasion heated debate as to the group decision for the appropriate avenue of care selected.

Already there is direct technological communication between individual educational centres across England, Wales and Northern Ireland, allowing for on-line discussion, knowledge transfer, information storage and retrieval as well as uploading and downloading of programs; in all an opportunity to reduce 'wheel reinvention' and a chance to go forward with a corporate voice through individual effort and communication. Included with the technological communication system is electronic mail for immediate letter exchange and electronic conferencing for local and national debate on professional topics.

The development of interactive audio and video is another area with wide and varied uses in the future. The use of such systems allows multiple media input in training and education packages. An interactive system involves the use of a computer linked to either a video (tape or laser disc) or an audio cassette system. Interactive video permits the user to sit at a keyboard and view visual material in the form of either still pictures or film with normal voice or other audio material. The scenario then displayed will form questions for the user and the response will determine other visual material to be shown following the outcome of decisions made in the answering of the questions. It is simulation to a high degree, already in use in many commercial organizations for specialist training with very encouraging results. Interactive video permits the user to make mistakes or push the system to its limits in a safe environment whilst viewing the outcome and most interactive video authors believe that this aids in 'reality' training. It has proved to be effective in terms of cost in most large commercial applications, such as the banking and commerce sectors.

Interactive audio also has a place in the future. Instead of pictorial representation, audio sound is used, not in the form of computer-synthesized voices, but actual spoken word, music or other audio output. In the past, much text has been displayed on the screen in computer education packages, which has often detracted from the effect of the package. With interactive audio, the amount of screen text is reduced and thus issues of communication skills can be addressed, such as intonation in speech. In some respects it permits the user to be more creative, in that a scene is painted in words. Just as the radio permits the user to make certain assumptions regarding the sounds and voices heard, so interactive audio permits the user freedom in determining the non-verbal elements involved in communication interaction.

We are all aware of the power of non-verbal communication, and indeed some authorities have suggested that the non-verbal element in our communication accounts for over 75% of all communication. Take this element away and the user has to listen and hear what is going on in order to make decisions. The use of interactive audio is cheaper than that of interactive video, it may not seem as immediately exciting, but the potential for use in nursing is immense.

Education is the key to the future in nursing use of computers, for as with many other movements in nursing, if the body of knowledge is present and that knowledge is sound, the ability to move forward will be found by those to whom such a move is most relevant, namely the nurses themselves. The body of knowledge should be information-led, not technology-led, for in reality the technology can look after itself; nursing's responsibility to itself is to determine its own information requirements, then find a suitable technological (or non-technological) solution to information integration.

Chapter Six

The way ahead

Has the computer anything to offer us; have we anything to offer computing? These two questions have been the focus for this book, and it may have gone some way towards answering them. The real answers however, are going to come from the nursing population itself, and they may not be fully realized for many years to come. Are we right to consider using computers in an environment that is so highly people-orientated? Do we see our future as that of keyboard operators? Is it necessary for nurses to become programmers? The questions still need to be addressed by us, but, in the light of the previous chapters, there should be reduced concern relating to the second and third points (keyboard operator/programmer). Indeed the answer to those two questions must be a considered 'No' for the majority of us.

Nursing's past role has not always been clear in the implementation process of computers and information technology in the hospital, community or education areas; perhaps now we have greater awareness of the need for nurses to be 'high-profile' in such developments as content experts.

We are all used to the growth of technology in health care, through computer-aided monitoring and the like, and such technological tools assist those involved in the care of patients and clients, often permitting extended life to those for whom we care. We are part of that technological growth and as such must not permit the essential understanding to pass us by at speed. The role of the nurse today, either in the community, hospital or in education, is now far more complex than for past generations of nurses. The essentials of care remain basically the same and justifiably so, but the addition (e.g. administrative duties and the drive for more qualifications, both practical and academic) can sap away our time from these essentials. If there is a tool available to help us, removing some of the time taken in the additional administrative aspects we should use it to the full.

Our responsibility is to ourselves, our patients, our colleagues and the future generations of nurses, and we must attend to these responsibilities in order to have an autonomous voice in the future. As the facilities of the technology increase, the uses in health care will similarly increase, if we wish that to be the case. Looking to the future is a very dangerous business and inherent within most of us is a design feature which does not permit accuracy when gazing into a crystal ball. Trends can be assumed from a base of discussions already taking place, and it is these trends that will be considered. Brief examination of the technological advances in computing in the near future may suggest many uses for this tool in health care.

TRENDS IN COMPUTER TECHNOLOGY

It is becoming increasingly evident that these developments generally involve three common elements:

1. smaller components;
2. faster delivery of service;
3. greater memory capacity.

The first is not only related to the actual computer itself, but also to its data storage medium. Currently available on the market are powerful lap-top computers, that can fit into a brief case. These often have large memory capacities that four years ago would have been considered as fairy tales. Some of the lap-top computers can be installed in cars and connected to the telephone system, similar to the in-car telephone system presently used, and this development is expected to be a boon for travelling sales people.

Hand-held computers, already available with full QWERTY keyboards and data storage and retrieval functions, are expected to become more powerful; in times to come owning one of these may outweigh the present use of paper time management systems.

As components get smaller, so the speed of information retrieval grows, due to the second two elements above; faster delivery of data and greater memory capacity. Increased memory capacity of computers does not always mean faster delivery of information, but with the development of reduced instruction set microprocessor (RISC) technology (where only the essential commands are examined by the computer) this certainly does seem to be the case. With RISC technology the microcomputer memory capacity is increased, in terms of working capacity internally (RAM), as is the speed in delivery of information within the system.

It would also appear that there is greater movement towards standardization in computer-to-computer communication, which has been assisted by the development of EC directives. Currently work is underway to align major computer systems to meet the standards set by the Open Systems Interchange (OSI) directives. The standards suggest seven elements to OSI ranging from the base of the number of bits transferred, to the more esoteric and technically advanced requirements for actual interchange between differing operating systems. Similarly, there appears to be a movement towards one computer being able to emulate others. For example, the Acorn Archimedes computer, running RISC technology, can emulate IBM or BBC BASIC or UNIX, each of which has a different operating environment. Due to the utilization of the RISC operating system, the machine can emulate others (with appropriate software) at a reasonable speed. Indeed, even IBM machines can emulate BBC BASIC with the use of a 'translation' software package.

The computer boom, having now lasted about seven years is showing some signs of slowing, especially in the home market. Sales are still high and no doubt will continue to be so for some time to come, but generally the reasons for purchase have changed, away from games towards home management and educational functions. There does seem to be a distinct movement away from the technology towards application software use by all.

Availability of application software is on the increase, and here the user need have no computing knowledge, but only requires a tool to manipulate and organize information. A growth in the use of spreadsheets, database tools and wordprocessing seems clear; it is possible that many of us could be called technocrats and that would be quite satisfactory, for technocrats use the tools at their disposal to their most effective levels, they are applications people if you like, and certainly we, as nurses need to count ourselves in this area, and soon.

NURSING'S TECHNOCRATIC FUTURE

An idea very slowly becoming reality, is that some hospital information computer systems have the nursing input as the central element, the linchpin upon which everything else hangs. Such developments are beginning to happen as nurses are seen as the health care professionals with the greatest day-to-day contact with patients or clients, the ward once again being the focal point around which all other departments operate. But it must said that this is not universal and indeed it would frequently appear as though the nursing section on a major computer system is thought of at a very late stage during information technology development within most hospital or community units.

It is unfortunate that to date most information technology developments have been viewed negatively by nurses, due in the main to their lack of involvement with such developments. Often the initial introduction nurses have is in information gathering for the new system, generally involving form completion in addition to their already pressurized working day. However, where nurses have been involved from early stages the picture tends to be considerably more optimistic.

Imagine, if you will, a nursing system based upon the identification of patient problems, aims of care, planning and implementation of care and evaluation of outcomes. The nurse in inputting the information triggers a number of other systems into operation, such as patient administration, theatre listing, laboratories, stores ordering, catering, transport, portering; the list goes on. All of this is activated through nurses carrying out their role and receiving information relevant to the nursing role. This is not a pipe dream; systems such as this are already in operation and more are on the way. A simple view of such an integration can be seen in Figure 6.1.

Growth in the area of communication through the use of technology will also become increasingly evident over forthcoming years. We have spoken earlier of the use of networking; imagine this on a national basis between different health disciplines. There will be a number of communication network systems to meet differing needs, and net-

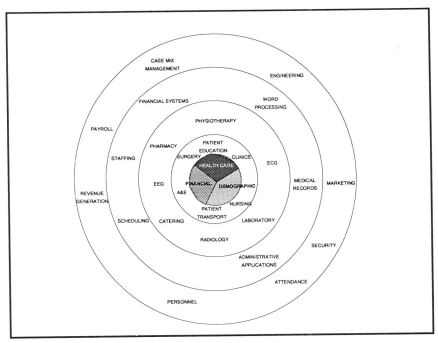

Figure 6.1 Diagrammatic representation of the information interrelationships within a major hospital computer system. The colour area represents the patient at the centre (Adapted from O'Desky, 1988).

worked general practitioner systems, aiding communication between different health centres are already in existence. The GPs using the system have found that there is a vast reduction in time in searching for notes, updating them and sending patient notes on to a new general practitioner. It is likely that the future will see a growth of such networks in community practice.

In nursing, wide area networking (WAN) through modem linkage will develop further, and such a communication network is already widely available in nursing and midwifery education. There are areas where communication networking could enhance current practice, such as the implementation of student nurse records transmission to a central computer rather than relying upon postal systems, providing a faster more efficient service to all concerned.

Another development making inroads into health care computer systems is the use of bar code input devices, whose use may most easily be described in the area of stock control and stores ordering, although it must be said that these are not the only potential uses. The items all have bar coding on them, just like many items currently in supermarkets or department stores, a laser pen is passed over the coding and the item is registered on a central computer. When stock is used, the bar code reading device is linked to an ordering computer and thus the stores computer can keep an accurate account of articles used. Within the stores computer would be information relating to what level is met before restocking is required, and in this way no stock ordering needs to be separately undertaken by the item user.

The bar code reading system has been tried in the clinical area for the input of patient information at the bedside. Core phrases were translated into bar codes and displayed upon a board, the user wishing to input information selected the phrase required, and through the use of a laser pen a direct link from the board transmitted the information to a computer. It is possible that the future may see greater use of this input device; indeed, commercially available computer systems for data collection at the bedside have included bar code readers in a hand-held device used by nurses, a system developed in the US. Part of the reason for the bar code system development is the belief that nurses should not have to learn how to type in order to input information; ease of use of computers and peripheral devices is the key for the future.

TECHNOLOGICAL DEVELOPMENTS FOR CONSIDERATION BY NURSES

In keeping with the belief that the user interface with computers should be as easy as possible, there has been a development of VDU touch screens, which are generally either light- or heat-sensitive. The computer screen displays items for choice, the user touches the area required with a finger or with a light-pen, and through a cascade system reaches the desired area without having to resort to a keyboard. The limitations of such a system is that only what is shown can be chosen, but if the system is adequately designed to meet a specific need this need not be a detrimental factor.

Voice-activated systems are in the very early stages of development, but it is likely that these will increase in effectiveness and use in forth-coming years. Present research is being undertaken in the area of word-processing where the user talks to the computer and the letter or document appears on the screen and, when required, in hard copy format. This could have potential uses for the disabled, especially as computers are already being found to be most beneficial both for those with physical handicaps and people with learning difficulties.

Output devices are also developing rapidly, perhaps one of the major breakthroughs in recent times being the laser printer. These devices remain costly, especially the Postscript ones, but with further modifications the cost is likely to decrease and such a printer may become available in many application areas. Already there are non-Postscript laser printers on the market at affordable prices. The power of such a printer is that it does not confine the user to text or schematic drawings. It permits a wide variety of hard copy displays on each sheet of paper; currently it is widely used in publication areas such as books, magazines, papers and information sheets.

Storage devices too are undergoing transformation for technology does not stand still. In the early days of computing there was not the ability to store information on floppy discs. Floppy discs are really quite a new occurrence and the first ones available on the market tended to be large, about 8 or 9 inches in diameter and of limited practical use outside a major computer installation. We are now used to seeing and using the 5¼ inch variety and more recent developments have brought the now-commonplace 3½ inch floppy disc with more storage than the 5¼ disc. The new floppy discs tend not to be 'floppy' in the recognized sense, in that the magnetic disc is surrounded by a hard plastic jacket thus permitting greater portability. Again the future will probably see a swing away from the 5¼ inch floppy disc to the 3½ inch more portable disc. The larger 5¼ inch disc will be with us for some time, but already most hardware manufacturers are producing computers with 3½ inch disc drives as standard.

The use of compact disc ROMs is also increasing, the disc resembling that of the audio compact disc available in record shops; with digitized input on to the disc both computer programs and pictures can be stored. Currently, compact disc (CD) ROMs are used in libraries holding vast amounts of text information. A use that is undergoing testing is that of picture libraries stored on CD-ROM. These pictures can be set up to meet specific demands, for example parts of complex engineering designs, medical anatomy, fabric patterns or electrical circuitry. Once the library is formed, users can 'call it up' and download into their own program the picture required, thus saving time and effort in trying to reproduce these difficult pictures. Another use being tried is that of storing information that tends to be static, such as national information on courses available at universities and polytechnics. The reason for the need to find static uses is that as yet a simple and cheap way of changing information held on CD-ROM has not been developed, but this is likely to change with the passage of time.

EXPERT SYSTEMS AND ARTIFICIAL INTELLIGENCE

It is almost impossible to keep track of the number of developments on the horizon and the above are just some of them to demonstrate the advances that are under way in the hardware area. Software developments are certainly not lagging behind and the two perhaps most constantly spoken about are 'expert systems' and 'artificial intelligence'.

An expert system is one that is built upon expertise and grows with use. For example, in the medical area to develop an expert system for use in the diagnosis of potential cardiology problems, a number of recognized authorities in the field would gather together and identify all their methods of assessment, including the type of questions they ask patients in order to form a diagnosis. All this information would be fed into a computer and the program would follow an 'IF-THEN' schedule. The following is a simplified version as in reality the number of variables may be many hundreds,

> IF the respondent states an age over 55
>
> and, IF the respondent states a weight over certain parameters set
>
> and, IF the respondent states a working environment likely to cause stress
>
> THEN certain other questions would be asked relating to greater in-depth responses
>
> and, IF the respondent answered these questions outside certain parameters
>
> THEN likely potential problems will be identified leading to diagnosis identification.

During use of the system, the computer 'learns' about new 'IF-THEN' areas and adds these to its memory for use during further questioning of respondents. When it comes upon something new or something it does not understand, the computer will ask the respondent how the new phrase differs from items already in its memory, thus trying to make comparisons between what is known to it and what is new. If the computer is satisfied that the new item is different enough from previous identified areas, the new area will be added to the 'IF' section. There is development under way for a nursing expert system, which is extremely exciting for our future, but the success of such a development requires understanding by the end user and hence our need to understand the present in order to play a part in the future.

The first stage in developing an expert system is that of forming a knowledge base. This base may be used as a bank of information to be examined, or as the basis for a logic to be assigned. If the base is used for the latter, the hard work is in preparing the logical sequence of the enquirer to the appropriate elements held on the knowledge base. It is suggested that specialist expertise is required for such logic setting, although an expert on the content must act in an advisory capacity.

Artificial intelligence is another kettle of fish. The phrase has often been quoted, but the reality at the moment is that no such system has yet been evolved. Many people associate it with sophisticated expert systems and indeed the development of expert systems would certainly appear to be the forerunner of artificial intelligence but the latter goes beyond that; quite where this author does not yet know, and researchers into this form of computer technology appear to be similarly unsure.

WHERE DOES NURSING GO NOW?

With these future developments, some almost upon us, has computing anything to offer us? The answer surely must be 'yes'; but more importantly, have we (the nurses) anything to offer computing? Again the answer must be 'yes', for we are the 'experts' in our own professional area and before we lose our identity altogether we must learn about the computer tool and harness it to our advantage before others harness it for us.

To repeat a subject from the first chapter, in a talk at the 1982 international conference, *The Impact of Computers on Nursing*, one speaker made a clear and easily understood point, and it is in some way sad that we have taken a period of ten years before the words have hit home.

'The choice is there and the time to make the choice is now. The decision must be whether to act traditionally and have change thrust upon the profession from the outside or to anticipate this revolution in nursing practice, familiarize nurses with it, and prepare them to take an active part in the introduction of computers into the nursing community.'

Berg, 1982

We must go forward and face the challenge offered to us by information technology and computers. We know our role, that of health care practitioner, but we must enhance the role through whatever means are at our disposal in order that we can continue to ensure adequate standards of patient and client care. We must also recognize the knowledge and skills of others and not attempt to take on board the whole world of computers and information technology; we must find our place in the team. Information understanding is the cornerstone of information technology development and frankly the technology can look after itself. Nursing must understand and be in control of information, for as stated at a recent conference,

'Power is control, influence or the ability to do or act. Power is the ability to make decisions and power is determining what those decisions will be in the first place. Power is having control of information.'

Gaston, 1991

The understanding of 'information' is a complex process, particularly when related to individuals, for each and every one of us is likely to view 'information' differently, and we all handle information in a different way. In order to carry out any activity, from waking in the morning to sleeping at night, we need and use vast amounts of information. We may not always think that we are using information, for some is so inbred that actions become automatic, but when we come to think about a name or place, our information system is consciously activated and we dig deep into our memory store to solve the information requirement.

'Information is the key to every activity of every one every day.'

Procter, 1991

If information is the key, what process does the key open to give power? Recently a diagrammatic representation of information handling was clearly given in Technocrat 12 (1991) and it is reproduced as Figure 6.2. More traditional views of the information process are linear and usually uni-directional: input to process to output. However, the radical representation of four engaging cogs as shown in Figure 6.2 is probably a more realistic model of the human information process, depicting the intertwining of the elements to form a rounded frame which is continually turning.

As shown in the cog diagram, information input is from two primary sources, value-laden (squiggly line) and bland (straight line). Almost all information we acquire has values placed upon it, either by an individual or organization through the way something is said, written or shown. Indeed, we ourselves place an immediate value on acquired information by deciding to retain or reject the new item.

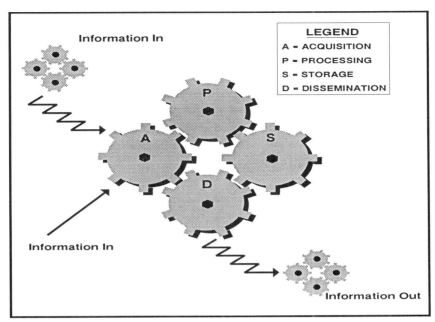

Figure 6.2 Diagrammatic representation of information flow (ENB CAL Project, 1991).

Every time we use our eyes, ears and noses or touch something, we take in information, some of which we accept without question, some of which we challenge and some of which we deeply question. For example, a common source of information is our own home where we are used to seeing certain treasured items in their allotted places; we generally accept the sight without question. What if we see a stain on the carpet, caused perhaps by a water leak? This is new information; we challenge it and determine the fault, correcting the fault ourselves if it is within our ability, or obtaining relevant assistance. How do we know how to mend the fault, how do we know what assistance we require, how do we know whom to call? Previously stored information is quickly retrieved to solve the problem. A friend telephones, and explains that they too have just found a similar problem in their home and they are not sure what course of action to take. It is more than likely that you now explain to your friend your solution, and in that way disseminate the information in a useful and appropriate way. All four cogs were interlinked, information was acquired, processed, stored and disseminated, not only by yourself, but also externally by your friend. Nursing practice information could be treated in exactly the same way as the 'home' example given; the individual information process remains the same. After all, what is the nursing process but an organized tool for information management? This includes:

1. information assessment of patient or client problems (potential and actual);
2. informed planning of care relative to the assessed problems;
3. competent implementation of care based upon informed and practiced methods;
4. structured evaluation and re-assessment based upon informed expected outcomes.

Nursing has a vast knowledge base derived from research and practice, which acts as an information base for accountable practitioners to use and adapt to meet individual patient or client requirements.

The same analysis and synthesis of information for use with technology must be forthcoming for nursing to survive in our current information-hungry society. As a recent Department of Health (1989) document states,

> 'Accountable practitioners, must be more than passive recipients of information. They will need to acquire the analytical skills to ask the right questions, to know where to seek answers to them, and to reach informed decisions on the basis of the fullest knowledge available.'

It is imperative that nurses do not bury their heads in the sand and hope that all the technology commotion goes away, for it will not. As Stonier (1981) stated,

> 'An educated workforce learns how to exploit new technology, an ignorant one becomes its victim.'

Nurses must come to terms with the developments in computers and information technology and become part of the growing practitioners in informatics. There has been a gradual development of nursing informatics since the late 1960s, but it was not until 1985 that the phrase 'nursing informatics' first came into being (Hannah, 1985). Even more recently the term has evolved; Graves and Corcoran (1989) state that nursing informatics is a,

> '. . . combination of computer science, information science and nursing science designed to assist in the management and processing of nursing data, information and knowledge to support the practice of nursing and the delivery of nursing care.'

Thus, we must combine our nursing knowledge with an understanding of the power of computers and information in order to remain at the forefront of health care delivery. As suggested earlier in this book, there is not a need to add computer programming or computer systems analysis to our role, but we owe it to ourselves and to our patients and clients to become aware of the technological tools to such a degree that we, as nurses, maintain control of the information that flows through these powerful tools.

Computers and information technology developments will have major influences in the way we deliver care, the way we manage health care and in the way we organize the supportive structure around the practical care delivery units. The impact has been well described in a World Health Organization publication *Informatics and Telematics in Health: Present and Potential Uses* (1988). It is pertinent here to cite a short section from the book's epilogue;

> 'Today, most institutions are compelled to assimilate new technology. Unlike many other innovations, however, the introduction of informatics technologies has a systematic impact on the entire organization. Introducing computers requires even more careful attention to change management compared to other technologies. Both structural and behavioural changes have to be considered. A strategy is required for both kinds of problems, and the implementation and monitoring of this strategy must be carefully managed. There is strong evidence that organizations which have successfully introduced informatics are more effective and efficient than those which have not attempted it or been unsuccessful in the transition.
>
> The computer itself will raise new social issues.'

The introduction of computers to a professional community is not a case of buying the hardware and software then expecting it all to evolve into effective working practice; there must be adequate education, training and understanding of the impact the 'boxes' will have within the health care community. This has often been under-considered or worse still, been ignored, leaving many nurses ignorant of the power of information technology.

Nursing must become involved in the health society changes as influenced by the introduction of computers and information technology. Indeed, according to the United Kingdom Central Council's (UKCC) *Code of Professional Conduct* (1988), nurses must,

> '. . . take every reasonable opportunity to maintain and improve professional knowledge and competence.'

Other disciplines within the health care sector are tackling the information technology revolution. Nursing too has made major steps forward in the use of computers to assess, deliver and support practice, but there remains a gulf between those few with knowledge and those, greater in number, with either limited or no knowledge of computers and information technology.

'The most successful health care delivery units of the future will be those where the main focus is on quality patient care. The factors essential for providing quality care are clinical expertise, systems to support comprehensive nursing and clinical data collection, ownership of information and good communications and working partnerships between disciplines.'

Thompson, 1991

What must never be forgotten in this dynamically developing health care society is nursing's base of clinical, community and educational knowledge. Such knowledge is paramount, but nursing must also open it's eyes and ears to the emerging discipline of informatics, embrace it and learn how to channel it towards increased professional competence and control.

We must do more than mechanize an organizational system where working practices have rarely been allowed fully to appraise changes that have been implemented locally or nationally. If we in the health care services are to develop information systems and computerize by integrating information systems, then let us do it well, with adequate organizational, managerial and educational support, and let us not pretend that by having a computer to carry out previous manual administrative tasks we have 'computerized'.

'In an increasingly computerized environment, power will belong to those who control information.'

Hales, 1988

The aim of this book is to give nurses confidence and an insight into computers and information technology, and to see where computers and information technology can fit into our present working practices without being detrimental to those working practices. The book, it is hoped, has raised questions in the reader's mind, questions to which answers may now be sought — certainly that was the intention.

A list is given of further reading should you wish to move beyond the limitations of this book.

Appendix A

Glossary

The following phrases or words are to be found in the text and they are commonly used when talking about computers or computing. The glossary attempts to clarify meanings for the reader but new words or phrases are continually coming into operation so when it doubt ask the user their meaning.

access time
The time taken to retrieve a piece of information from (usually) secondary storage.

A/D
An abbreviation for analogue to digital. It refers to the two types of 'signal' used in computers and related data transmission facilities.

algorithm
A set of instructions that enables a particular problem to be solved.

analogue/analog
A physical continuous signal as distinct from a digital discrete representation of a signal.

ANSI
An acronym for the American National Standards Institute whose brief is to formulate guidelines on computing standards.

archive
Store files off-line to make room for new input and to keep the system running efficiently.

ASCII
American Standard Code for Information Interchanging. A widely used computer code for the representation of characters within a computer system. It allows for some standardization between manufacturers in the structure of their systems, in that files stored in ASCII form can be transferred between computers, particularly through a communication network.

backlog
All work in a computer environment must be scheduled for processing in an orderly and acceptable manner. For many reasons, disruption will occur which causes the workflow to deviate from the designed schedule. Unprocessed work resulting from these deviations is termed backlog.

back-up
An additional copy of a file stored on another disc or a duplicate of a complete disc. Also used as a term for tape storage for major computer systems.

bar code
Codes of bars, each of varying thickness which are used to represent data

bar code reader
Device based upon optical or magnetic principles which recognizes the patterns comprising the code and converts the data into a form usable by the computer.

BASIC
An acronym for Beginner's All-purpose Symbolic Instructional Code, a computer language developed originally in 1964 in the USA for beginners to programming computers. It is a powerful language that is relatively easy to use.

batch
A term originating from traditional computer systems whereby work submitted to the computer had to be prepared in sets. Such batches would be processed in one single operation.

Baud
Used to describe the rate of transfer of information per second. It refers to the transfer of individual bits. A transfer rate of 1200 Baud = 120 characters per second.

binary
The language of computers. Circuits can only be either open or closed, that is with the current flowing or not flowing, and information is represented using binary patterns (see bit).

bit	(Binary digITS) The smallest unit of representation which a computer will recognize and use within its circuitry. Each bit has two possible values '0' or '1', frequently corresponding to a closed or open circuit.
bubble memory	Data/information which is stored on several magnetically charged crystal chips.
bug	The jargon for a fault or error within the program.
byte	A group of 8 'bits' strung together to represent a number or character.
catalog	A list of the contents of a disc.
central processing unit (CPU)	The part of the computer which performs computations, reads, interprets and processes information, oversees the use of the main memory and controls the input and output operations of the system.
centronics interface	An industry-compatible system for passing data from the computer to a printer or other output device.
channel	Describes the logical connection for communication purposes, from the CPU of a system to its input and output devices.
chip	A rectangular wafer of silicon upon which intricate circuitry is built layer by layer.
COBOL	A programming language. It stands for COmmon Business Orientated Language and was developed to process business applications.
computer	A general-purpose machine capable of carrying out any task defined by a set of instructions.
concurrent operation	Simultaneous operation with two or more workstations inputting data at the same time when sharing a CPU and hard disc.

configuration   An arrangement of computer system components.

CP/M   Control Programming for Microcomputers, a popular operating system.

cursor   A flashing or solid rectangle or horizontal line which indicates on the VDU the position of the next typed character.

data   Raw facts and figures.

database   An organized pool of data.

data processing   The processing of raw data to produce ordered, meaningful information. This term does not, and indeed should not imply the use of a computer.

dedicated machine   Implies that the machine concerned is reserved for either one user or one type of application.

destination disc   The disc to which a file is being copied from another disc.

digital   The discrete representation of information in contrast to the analogue representation used for some applications.

disc drive   The mechanism which spins the disc at a high speed and rapidly reads information from it or writes information to it using a magnetic head.

DOS   Abbreviation for Disc Operating System.

dot matrix   Characters on the screen are made of dots and the arrangement of the dots in a given area is called the dot matrix. The more dots in a dot matrix the clearer the character or picture. Also referred to in printers.

double density discs   Generally applied to floppy discs and reflects an increased capacity for storage.

double-sided discs Another means of increasing the storage capacity of a floppy disc. Files can be stored on both sides of the disc and a suitable disc drive is required to read and write to both sides.

down time The period during which the system is inoperable.

dumb terminal A terminal, usually a VDU and keyboard, that lacks its own CPU, secondary storage and printer. Should the central resource fail, the terminal ceases to function.

dump The storing of data on to another medium. For example, from screen to printer or disc.

EDP Electronic data processing defines processing as being effected by electronic (i.e. computing) methods.

electronic mail The electronic transmission of documents from one device to another, usually referred to when using wide area communications networks, but also using in-house local area networks.

EPROM Erasable Programmable Read Only Memory. A chip-based data storage facility.

ergonomics The study of fitting the equipment to the operator with emphasis on safety, comfort and efficiency.

execute Taken to mean the initiation of some action.

external storage Also known as secondary memory, back-up memory, long-term storage. It is complementary to the main memory of the computer system.

field In data organization a field is an item of data. Several fields or items of related data make up a record.

file A group of similar records kept together.

firmware   Used to describe software supplied by the
                        manufacturer of the system which is physically
                        incorporated into the computer system's
                        design. Can also be used to describe a piece
                        of hardware with software embedded on to it
                        permanently.

floppy disc   Recording medium on which information is
                        stored, generally magnetic.

font   Describes the range of characters (the character
                        set) which a printer is able to produce.

format   The task of preparing a disc in order that infor-
                        mation can be stored upon it. The format pro-
                        cess is essentially the same for all computers,
                        but once a disc is prepared for a particular
                        machine or operating system, in general terms
                        it cannot be used with a different machine or
                        operating system type.

formatted disc   A disc which has been prepared to accept (store)
                        files.

FORTRAN   Acronym for FORmula TRANslator, a high-
                        level programming language developed in the
                        mid–1950s. It is mathematically orientated and
                        is largely used for scientific and engineering
                        applications.

function keys   These are keys which are designed to initiate a
                        particular action specific to the job being
                        worked upon.

GIGO   An abbreviation for 'garbage in, garbage out'.
                        The phrase is used to illustrate the complete
                        dependence of computer systems upon accurate
                        input of data.

hard copy   The paper copy of a processed document or file.

hard disc   This is the larger, more powerful version of
                        random access secondary storage media, the
                        smaller alternative being the floppy disc.

hardware	The tangible (or physical) parts of a computer system, i.e. all input and output devices.
high-level language	A computer language close to that of natural human language, for example BASIC.
high resolution	Quality of graphics display on the screen or printer in great detail and to a high degree of accuracy.
IC	An abbreviation of integrated circuit.
icons	Pictures or symbols used on the screen to represent files, documents, in/out trays, etc.
IEEE/IEEE–488	A type of communication between a computer and its printer.
information	Information refers to the ordered selected and sorted facts and figures that are meaningful to the user. Data are thus processed to become information.
initialized	For a disc, this is synonymous with the term 'formatted'.
input	Data or text entered into the computer system.
integrated software	Software that allows the operator to perform complicated tasks involving the use of more than one application without the need to stop and change discs.
interface	In computing, this term refers to an electro-mechanical link between individual components of the system.
ISO standard	The official European name for ASCII code.
K	Abbreviation taken to mean 1000. (For the technically minded, K = 1024 for computing applications.)
load	The transference of a program or of data into the computer's memory.

low-level language   A computer language near to the computer's own binary language of 0 and 1; for example machine code.

light pen   A device which the user points at the screen to select an activity or draw the input.

magnetic media   A generic term for cards, discs, cassettes, etc.

mainframe   Usually refers to a large computer installation, in contrast to mini or micro systems.

megabyte   A unit of measurement representing one million bytes.

memory   There are two categories of memory, internal and external. Internal memory is stored within the computer whilst work is in progress (RAM) but is generally lost when the computer is turned off. External or secondary memory provides the storage facilities whereby completed files can be saved and retrieved when required.

microcomputer   A computer that is small in size and driven by a microprocessor.

microprocessor   Carries out all of the arithmetic and logic functions of the system in addition to its overall controlling function.

minicomputer   Between mainframe and microcomputer in size.

modem   An abbreviation of MOdulator/DEModulator. It enables data to be transmitted across ordinary telephone lines so that one computer can 'talk' to another computer, through translating computer (binary) signals into telephone (analog) signals and back again.

monitor   A VDU screen, some of which are now capable of transmitting video as well as displaying information as an output device to the CPU.

mouse	A hand-held pointing device which is used to input commands and quickly move the cursor across the screen.
natural language	Languages as spoken by people.
network	A facility which interconnects all the electronic equipment in a building (local area network), or across telephone lines and computer lines (wide area network) so that communication and sharing of information can take place.
off-line storage	Storage of files on discs or tapes which are not under the direct control of the CPU.
on-line storage	Discs, tapes, etc. under the direct control of the CPU (i.e. in the disc drive).
operating system	A collection of programs that controls the operation of other external programs and application software.
output	The end product of a computer operation.
parallel interface	Method of passing information from the computer to its printer or output device.
password	Access code to a system, usually found in large systems where confidentiality is paramount.
peripherals	Attachments to the CPU, e.g. keyboard, VDU, disc drives, printer, mouse, etc.
pixel	The basic element of a VDU's image. Each character on a screen is composed of a defined number of pixels.
port	A technical term referring to a socket, sometimes called a slot or channel.
PRESTEL	Public viewdata system, accessible through a wide area communications network.
primary sort	Sorting in the first order of priority.

program   A set of instructions which tells the computer what to do, step by step.

PROM   Programmable Read Only Memory, a silicon ROM chip whose contents may be altered by the user.

protected field   A portion of data that cannot be modified directly by the operator.

protocols   Rules and conventions for transmitting data.

purge   Erase files from discs.

query languages   Languages that have been compiled especially for management to question a system's database.

QWERTY keys   Standard typewriter key set.

random access   Refers to a method of retrieving information within a computer system, usually from the secondary memory.

RAM   Random Access Memory, also referred to as the internal working memory.

real-time   A system that is able to respond immediately to changes made in its database.

response time   The time required to retrieve or process data or text.

RF modulator   A device which encodes a composite video signal into a radio-frequency signal display on a standard television.

ROM   Read Only Memory. Information contained within a silicon chip which, once created, cannot be amended or changed in any way.

RS232/RS423   A method of passing data between the com-
Interface   puter and usually a modem. The serial interface is sometimes used.

sector	A contiguous section of a disc track. A block of data is identified by its unique track and sector number.
sequential access	Involves the retrieval of information by reading the items, one by one, from the beginning of the document or file. Generally tape, and generally slow.
serial interface	A method of transferring data from a wordprocessor to its printer. Contrasts with parallel-based interfaces.
single density	Term used to denote that the storage of information within a medium such as disc is not compressed in any way.
soft copy	Intangible output on the VDU.
software	In its broadest sense, software refers to the programs which provide the driving force of all computing systems. There are two basic kinds; operating systems software and applications software.
source disc	The disc on which a file to be copied is stored.
stand alone	The computer system is designed in such a way that it requires no additional material, software or hardware to be effective.
system	A group of interacting parts that operate together to achieve a common goal.
system disc	The disc on which the operating system is stored.
systems analyst	A computer professional whose job is to analyse the existing system or function and design an efficient computerized system to meet the required need.
topology	A term used to define the shape of a network.

turnaround time   Time taken to produce a completed file or document from receipt of the original draft.

user friendly   Term to describe a system that is designed to be easy to use.

user interface   Devices and methods incorporated in hardware
technology   and software which allow the user to think and act intuitively, thus making computers easier to use.

utility programs   Service programs that perform certain actions pertaining to the system in use at that time, such as disc formatting.

VDU   Abbreviation for visual display unit.

windows   The display of more than one document on the screen at one time, allowing the user to take information from one document or file and insert it into another.

workstation   A connected keyboard and VDU at which the operator works.

Appendix B

The Data Protection Act — 1984

Computers are in use throughout society, collecting, storing, processing and distributing information. Much of that information is about people — personal data — and is now subject to the Data Protection Act.

The Act aims to protect personal data by establishing and enforcing certain standards for data processing. It also enables the United Kingdom to ratify the Council of Europe's Convention on Data Protection, ensuring that data flows freely and safely between the United Kingdom and other European countries.

This appendix offers some guidance to data users about their obligations under the Act, and it attempts to answer some of the questions which are commonly asked, but the information given below should not be regarded as offering a definitive statement on the Act. More guidance is available from the Data Protection Officer within your local Health Authority or Trust.

PROTECTING PERSONAL DATA

The Data Protection Act will affect most of us either as data users or data subjects through,

- the establishment of a public register of **DATA USERS**
- the creation of an independent **DATA PROTECTION REGISTRAR** with special powers to ensure that personal data are processed in accordance with the **EIGHT DATA PROTECTION PRINCIPLES** (see later)
- the setting up and maintenance of a **DATA PROTECTION TRIBUNAL**
- the introduction of new rights for **DATA SUBJECTS**
- imposing certain obligations upon **DATA USERS**.

DATA USERS are people (often corporate bodies) who control the contents and use of automatically processed personal data. Unless exempted (see Exemptions) they have to register under the Act and comply with the data protection principles.

DATA SUBJECTS are individuals about whom information is held on computer. They have a new right of access to that information; entitled to have it corrected or erased in certain circumstances, and entitled to compensation if they suffer damage because data are inadequately protected, or inaccurate.

PERSONAL DATA is information held on computer about living, identifiable individuals, including expression of opinions about them.

NEW RIGHTS AND OBLIGATIONS

The Data User

What must I do to comply with the Act?

FIRST you must register. Failure to do so is a criminal offence. (Remember — not only your company/hospital, but you as an individual manager, secretary, teacher, clinician or similar officer may be liable to prosecution.)

SECOND, you must comply with the data protection principles and make sure that you do not do anything which is not covered by your register entry: operating outside the terms of your register entry will also be an offence. (You may, of course, amend your register entry if necessary by applying to the Registrar and may act as if your application had been accepted as soon as you have sent it.)

How Do I Register?

By applying to the Registrar and providing:

- [ ] your name and address (and hospital/department/college address)
- [ ] a description of the data you hold and the purposes for which you hold it
- [ ] description of sources, and recipients of your data (that is, persons to whom you disclose data) and countries to which you transfer data
- [ ] an address to which data subjects may write for access to their data.

You may make several entries in the register. If you hold large amounts of data for different purposes you may find it easier to register the different purposes separately. This may make it easier for you to deal with requests for access (which must relate to separate register entries) but you will have to pay a separate fee for each application.

More guidance is available from the Registrar.

To Whom May I Disclose Data?

Generally only to those people you have described in your register entry, and to the data subject. Disclosure to anyone else will usually be an offence (but see Exemptions).

Subject Access

If any individual enquires in writing whether you as a data user hold personal data about him/her, you must tell him/her, and you must provide him/her with a copy of the data (unless the exemptions apply).

Correction or Erasure

Data subjects are entitled to have inaccurate details, or data which are held in breach of any of the data protection principles, corrected or erased.

EXEMPTIONS

There are three categories of exemption, from the Act as a whole, from subject access and from the restrictions on disclosure of data.

Total Exemptions

The following categories of data are completely exempt from the Act (but remember – some of these exemptions are conditional – you must be sure that you comply with the conditions if you take advantage of an exemption),

- □ data held for national security purposes, data held ONLY for payroll and accounting purposes (BUT they must not be used for any other purpose and there are restrictions on disclosure)
- □ data required by law to be made publicly available by the user
- □ data held ONLY for the purpose of preparing the text of documents (e.g. wordprocessor)
- □ mailing lists consisting ONLY of names and addresses and data held by unincorporated clubs about their members (BUT only if the data subjects have been asked and have not objected and restrictions on disclosure are complied with) data held ONLY for domestic and recreational purposes.

Subject Access Exemptions

Subject access need not be given to data in the following categories:

☐ data held for law enforcement and revenue purposes, if access to them would be likely to prejudice those purposes

☐ data held by certain bodies for regulating those who provide financial services

☐ legally privileged data (data relating to judicial appointments)

☐ back-up data (i.e. data held in case the current data on the computer is lost or corrupted)

☐ data held only for statistics or research, if never used or disclosed for any other purpose and if the results are never made available in a form which identifies individuals.

In addition, the Secretary of State may make an order, either exempting from subject access data about physical or mental health and social work, or making special arrangements for granting access to such data.

Disclosure Exemptions

DATA CAN BE DISCLOSED IF

☐ the disclosure is for law enforcement or revenue purposes, if having to describe the recipient in the register entry would prejudice those matters

☐ the disclosure is for national security purposes

☐ the disclosure is required by law or by the order of a court or in legal proceedings.

☐ the data subject has consented to the disclosure

☐ the disclosure is required to be made urgently to prevent injury or damage to health.

EIGHT PRINCIPLES OF DATA PROTECTION

These principles are internationally agreed and form part of Schedule 1 of the Act. They require personal data to be,

1. obtained fairly and lawfully
2. held only for one or more lawful purpose specified in the data users' register entry
3. used or disclosed only in accordance with the data users' register entry
4. adequate, relevant and not excessive for those purposes
5. accurate and where necessary up to data
6. not kept longer than necessary for the specified purposes

7. made available to data subjects on request
8. properly protected against loss or disclosure.

WHERE CAN I OBTAIN FURTHER ADVICE?

A number of representative organizations have already prepared guidance for their members and some more general guidelines are available. For more details, contact your local Data Protection Act Officer.

References

Ball, M. J. and Hannah, K. J. (1984) *Using Computers in Nursing*, Reston Publishing, Virginia, USA.

Barber, B. (1983) Computers need nursing, in *The Impact of Computers on Nursing*, (eds M. Scholes, Y. Bryant and B. Barber) Elsevier Science Publishers B.V., pp. 24–33.

Barr, A. (1967) *Measurement of Nursing Care*, OR Research Unit Publication 9, Oxford Regional Health Board.

Berg, C. M. (1983) The importance of nurses' input for the selection of computerized systems, in *The Impact of Computers on Nursing*, (eds M. Scholes, Y. Bryant and B. Barber) Elsevier Science Publishers B.V., pp. 42–58.

Department of Health (1989) *A Strategy for Nursing: A Report of the Steering Committee*, chaired by Mrs A. Poole, Nursing Division, London.

English National Board for Nursing, Midwifery and Health Visiting Computer Assisted Learning Project (ENB CAL Project) (1991) Curriculum integration proposal document', addition to *The Technocrat*, Number 12, March.

Gaston, C. F. (1991) The politics of nursing information systems and resource allocation, in *Nursing Informatics '91* (eds E. J. S. Horenga, K. J. Hannah, K. A. McCormick and J. S. Ronald) Springer-Verlag, New York, pp. 3–13.

Graves, J. R. and Corcoran, S. (1989) The study of nursing informatics, *Image: Journal of Nursing Scholarship*, **21**, 227–31.

Hales, G. D. (1988) Computers in continuing education, in *Nursing Informatics, Where Caring and Technology Meet* (eds. M. J. Ball, K. J. Hannah, U. Gerdin *et al.*), Springer-Verlag, New York, pp. 344–50.

Hannah, K. J. (1985) Current trends in nursing informatics: implications for curriculum planning, in *Nursing Uses of Computers and Information Science*, (eds K. J. Hannah, E. J. Guillemin and N. Conklin) North-Holland, Amsterdam.

James, M. P. (1991) IT local strategies, in *The Technocrat*, ENB CAL Project Newsletter, March.

Körner, E. (1982) *A report on the collection and use of information about hospital clinical activity in the National Health Service: the steering group on health services information*, Her Majesty's Stationery Office, London.

Körner, E. (1984) *A report on the collection and use of information about hospital clinical activity in the National Health Service: the steering group on health services information*, Her Majesty's Stationery Office, London.

NHS Management Board Information Advisory Group (1986) *A National Strategic Framework for Information Management in the Hospital and Community Health Services*, Department of Health, London.

NHS Review (1989) *Working For Patients*, Department of Health, London.

O'Desky, R. I. (1988) A neural view of computing for nurses, in *Nursing Informatics, Where Caring and Technology Meet*, (eds. M. J. Ball, K. J. Hannah, U. Gerdin *et al.*) Springer-Verlag, New York, pp. 33–45.

Papert, S. (1980) *Mindstorms, Children, Computers and Powerful Ideas*, Harvester Press, London.

Procter, P. M. (1991) A national strategy for educational nursing informatics, in *Nursing Informatics in New Zealand: An Impetus for Learning*, (eds J. Hausman *et al.*), Conference Proceedings, pp. 135–42.

Redmond, D. T. (1983) An overview of the development of National Health Service computing, in *The Impact of Computers on Nursing*, (eds. M. Scholes, Y. Bryant and B. Barber) Elsevier Science Publishers B.V., pp. 59–69.

Roberts, R. and Taylor, J. A. (1987) Computerised clinical nursing information systems', in *Current Perspectives in Health Computing*, (eds. J. R. Bryant *et al.*), British Journal of Health Care Computing Books, pp. 196–202.

Stonier, T. (1981) Changes in western society — Educational implications, in *Recurrent Education and Lifelong Learning*, (eds. T. Sculler *et al.*), Kogan Page, London.

Thompson, J. M. E. (1991) The Northern Ireland perspective on nursing and computers, in *Nursing Informatics '91*, (eds E. J. S. Hovenga, K. J. Hannah, K. A. McCormick and J. S. Ronald) Springer-Verlag, New York, pp. 507–11.

United Kingdom Central Council for Nurses, Midwives and Health Visitors (1988) *Code of Professional Conduct*, UKCC, London.

Warne, B. E. M. (1983) Community nursing information systems, in *The Impact of Computers on Nursing*, (eds M. Scholes, Y. Bryant and B. Barber) Elsevier Science Publishers B.V., pp. 200–6.

World Health Organisation (1988) *Informatics and Telematics in Health: Present and Potential Uses*, WHO, Switzerland.

Further reading

COMPUTER BOOKS

Bradbeer, R., de Bono, P. and Laurie, P. (1982) *The Computer Book — an introduction to computers and computing*, British Broadcasting Corporation, London.

Dean, C. and Whitlock, Q. (1983) *A Handbook of Computer-Based Training*, Kogan Page, London.

Fulk, J. and Steinfield, C. (eds) (1990) *Organisations and Communications Technology*, SAGE Publications, Newbury Park, California.

Mathias, H., Rushby, N. and Budgett, R. (eds) (1988) *Aspects of Educational Technology XXI, Designing New Systems and Technologies for Learning*, Kogan Page, London.

Mullins, E. (1985) *Information Processing*, Pitman Publications.

Papert, S. (1980) *Mindstorms, Children, Computers and Powerful Ideas*, Harvester Press, London.

Wetherbe, J. C. (1979) *Systems Analysis for Computer-Based Information Systems*, West Publishing Company, St. Paul, Minnesota.

NURSING-RELATED COMPUTER BOOKS

Ball, M. J., Hannah, K. J., Gerdin Jelger, U., and Peterson, H. (eds) (1988) *Nursing Informatics. Where Caring and Technology Meet*, Springer-Verlag, New York.

Barber, B., Cao, D., Qin, D. and Wagner, G. (eds) (1989) *Proceedings of the Sixth Conference on Medical Informatics, MEDINFO 89*, Elsevier, Amsterdam.

Bryant, J. and Kostrewski, B. (eds) (1985) *Current perspectives in Health Computing 1985*, British Computer Society, London

Bryant, J., Roberts, J. and Windsor, P. (eds) (1987) *Current Perspectives in Health Computing 1987*, British Computer Society, London.

Cox, H. C., Harsany, B., and Dean, L. C. (1987) *Computers and Nursing — Application to Practice, Education and Research*, Appleton & Lange, East Norwalk, Connecticut.

Duigan, K. (1990) *Introduction to Information Management and Technology*, NHS Training Authority, Bristol (part of the Health PickUp Series).

de Glanville, H. and Roberts, J. (eds) (1990) *Current Perspectives in Health Computing 1990*, British Computer Society, London.

Greenhalgh and Co. Ltd *Nurse Management Systems, A Guide to Existing and Potential Systems*, Healthcare Management Consultants, Grasmere House, 38 Grasmere, Macclesfield, Cheshire, SK11 8PL.

Grobe, S. J. (1984) *Computer Primer and Resource Guide for Nurses*, Lippincott, Philadelphia, Pennsylvania.

Hovenga, E. J. S., Hannah, K. J., McCormick, K. A. and Ronald, J. S. (eds) (1991) *Nursing Informatics '91 — Proceedings of the Fourth International Conference on Nursing Use of Computers and Information Science*, Springer-Verlag, New York.

Koch, B. and Rankin, J. (eds) (1987) *Computers and their applications in Nursing*, Harper & Row, London.

Lochhaas, T. (ed) (1988) *Nursing and Computers. Third International Symposium on Nursing Use of computers and Information Science*, C. V. Mosby.

Mackay, G. and Griffin, A. (eds) *Nurses Using Computers, Australian Experiences*, ACAE Publications.

NHS Training Authority (1990) *Guide to Installation of Nursing Information Systems (GINIS)*, NHS Training Authority, Bristol.

Procter, P., Dowglass, M., Norman, S. and Vigar, T. (eds) (1991) *Working IT Together, ENB CAL Project Conference Proceedings*, ENB Publication.

Rowley, D. and Purser, H. (1988) *Clinical Information Technology: A practical guide to personal computing for healthcare clinicians and managers*, Taylor & Francis, London.

Scholes, M., Bryant, Y. and Barber, B. (eds) (1983) *The Impact of Computers on Nursing, an International Review*, North-Holland, Amsterdam.

Simons, P. (1990) *Using Information to Manage Resources*, NHS Training Authority, Bristol (part of the Health PickUp Series).

Smith, J. (1990) *Specifying and Collecting Information*, NHS Training Authority, Bristol (part of the Health PickUp Series).

Snook, R., Wright, G. and Brookman, P. (eds) (1988) *Proceedings of the Second National Conference on the use of Computers in Health Care Education and Training*, NHS Training Authority, Bristol.

Starling, P. (sub-ed) (1988) *Current Perspectives in Health Computing 1988*, British Computer Society, London.

Stewart, J. and Wood, W. (1990) *Using Information for Patient Care*, NHS Training Authority, Bristol (part of the Health PickUp Series).

Turley, J. P. and Newbold, S. K. (eds) (1991) *Nursing Informatics '91 — Pre-conference Proceedings*, Springer-Verlag.

Wright, G. and Brookman, P. (eds) (1986) *Proceedings of the First National*

Conference on the use of Computers in Health Care Education and Training, NHS Training Authority, Bristol.

Walker, M. B. and Schwartz, C. (1984) *What every Nurse should know about Computers*, Lippincott, Philadelphia, Pennsylvania.

World Health Organisation (1988) *Informatics and Telematics in Health — Present and Potential Uses*, WHO, Switzerland.

EDUCATION-RELATED COMPUTER BOOKS

Harris, D. (ed) (1988) Education for the new technologies in *World Yearbook of Education*, Kogan Page, London.

O'Shea, T. and Self, J. (1983) *Learning and Teaching with Computers — Artificial Intelligence in Education*, The Harvester Press, London.

Percival, F., Craig, D. and Buglass, D. (eds) (1987) *Flexible Learning Systems*, Kogan Page, London.

Rushby, N. and Howe, A. (eds) (1986) *Educational, Training and Information Technologies — Economics and Other Realities*, Kogan Page, London.

Tucker, J. (ed) (1984) *Education, Training and the New Technologies*, Kogan Page, London.

Index

Numbers in bold refer to figures